Essential Nursing Skills

Commissioning Editor: **Ninette Premdas**
Development Editor: **Fiona conn**
Project Manager: **Elouise Ball**
Designer: **Charlotte Murray**
Illustrator: **Cactus**
Illustration Manager: **Merlyn Harvey**

Essential Nursing Skills

THIRD EDITION

MAGGIE NICOL
BSc(Hons) MSc PGDipEd RN
Professor of Clinical Skills

CAROL BAVIN
DipN(Lond) RCNT RN RM

PATRICIA CRONIN
BSc(Hons) MSc(Nursing) DipN(Lond) RN
Senior Lecturer

KAREN RAWLINGS-ANDERSON
BSc(Hons) MSc(Nursing) DipNEd RN
Senior Lecturer

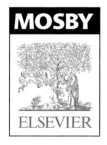

EDINBURGH LONDON NEW YORK OXFORD PHILADELPHIA ST LOUIS SYDNEY TORONTO 2008

MOSBY
ELSEVIER

An imprint of Elsevier Limited

© 2008, Elsevier Limited. All rights reserved.

First edition 2000
Second edition 2004
Third edition 2008

ISBN: 9780723434740

British Library Cataloguing in Publication Data
A catalogue record for this book is available from the British Library

Library of Congress Cataloging in Publication Data
A catalog record for this book is available from the Library of Congress.

Notice
Knowledge and best practice in this field are constantly changing. As new research and experience broaden our knowledge, changes in practice, treatment and drug therapy may become necessary or appropriate. Readers are advised to check the most current information provided (i) on procedures featured or (ii) by the manufacturer of each product to be administered, to verify the recommended dose or formula, the method and duration of administration, and contraindications. It is the responsibility of the practitioner, relying on their own experience and knowledge of the patient, to make diagnoses, to determine dosages and the best treatment for each individual patient, and to take all appropriate safety precautions. To the fullest extent of the law, neither the Publisher nor the Authors assumes any liability for any injury and/or damage to persons or property arising out of or related to any use of the material contained in this book.

The Publisher

ELSEVIER your source for books, journals and multimedia in the health sciences
www.elsevierhealth.com

Working together to grow libraries in developing countries
www.elsevier.com | www.bookaid.org | www.sabre.org

ELSEVIER | BOOK AID International | Sabre Foundation

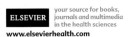

The publisher's policy is to use paper manufactured from sustainable forests

Printed in China

Contents

Preface

Why this book?

As nurse teachers who teach clinical skills to undergraduate nursing students and newly qualified nurses, we wanted to write a book that detailed how to perform the skills and could serve as a reminder for the skills they had been taught but may not have had an opportunity to practise for several weeks, maybe months. The book is designed to be small enough to carry around, especially when in clinical practice. The practice of nursing is dynamic and rapidly changing. This third edition has been thoroughly updated to reflect new guidelines and nursing practices.

What is it?

This book deliberately focuses on the skills required by nurses caring for adult patients in a hospital setting, but the skills themselves can be adapted to any clinical setting. It is a manual of skills that are essential to nursing: a 'how-to-do-it' book. It is not a textbook and so does not include all the theory and rationale that underpins the various skills, but suggestions for further reading are provided at the end of each chapter. Most skills are accompanied by 'Points for practice', a section that provides hints, suggestions or explanations to ensure successful performance of the skill.

The focus is on the practical aspects rather than why the skill is necessary. For example, insertion of a nasogastric tube explains how to select, measure and insert the tube; it does not discuss the reasons why such a tube may be necessary. This book is designed to complement nursing textbooks, not replace them.

How do I use it?

Each skill first describes preparation of the patient, the environment and the nurse, and the equipment needed. This is followed by a step-by-step description of the procedure, supported by illustrations, and additional information in the 'Points for practice'. The care required following the skill is then described. *Essential Nursing Skills* is designed to act as a reminder for skills that you have been taught, and to enable you to prepare yourself for new skills. *As with all aspects of nursing, it is vital that a Registered Nurse supervises you until you have really mastered each skill and are competent to carry them out alone.*

Nursing practice is subject to many local policies and protocols and the reader is reminded to refer to them throughout. Local policies and protocols refer to specific aspects of nursing practice that may vary between hospitals and include: drug-checking procedures (e.g. intravenous drug therapy); which nurses are permitted to perform the skill (e.g. male catheterisation); which dressing should be used (e.g. care of an intravenous cannula); the way equipment should be cleaned (e.g. dressing trolley); and the disposal of clinical waste. Notes pages have been included to enable you to make a note of relevant local policies and procedures.

We hope that you will find this book interesting, enjoyable and a valuable resource to support and enhance your clinical practice.

London, 2008

Maggie Nicol
Carol Bavin
Patricia Cronin
Karen Rawlings-Anderson

Acknowledgement

The authors would like to acknowledge the valuable contribution by Shelagh Bedford-Turner to the first two editions of this book.

1

Observation and monitoring

TEMPERATURE RECORDING

Preparation

Patient	Equipment/Environment	Nurse
• Explain procedure, to gain consent and co-operation.	• Disposable chemical thermometer, e.g. TempaDot PFP2 PFP3.	• Hands must be clean.
• Assess patient regarding suitable site for temperature recording PFP1.	• Observation chart.	• Additional protective clothing may be necessary if indicated by the patient's condition (see Chapter 9).
• Patient should not have had a hot or cold drink, smoked a cigarette within the previous 15 minutes when using the oral site.		

Procedure

Oral

1. Ask the patient to open their mouth, and gently insert the thermometer under their tongue, next to the frenulum PFP1. This is adjacent to a large artery (sublingual artery), so the temperature will be close to core temperature (Figure 1.1A).

2. Ask the patient to close their lips, but not their teeth, around the thermometer, to prevent cool air circulating in the mouth.

3. It is vital to leave the thermometer in position for the recommended length of time (usually 1 minute). However, it does not affect accuracy if it is left for longer than the minimum time.

4. Remove the thermometer, taking care not to touch the part that has been in the patient's mouth. In accordance with the manufacturer's instructions, read the temperature by noting the way that the dots have changed colour (see Figure 1.1C).

Axilla

1. Ask/assist the patient to expose their axilla. For an accurate recording, the axilla must be dry and free from sweat.

2. With the dots facing the chest wall, position the thermometer vertically between the arm and the chest wall and ask/assist the patient to keep their arm close against the chest to ensure good contact with the skin (see Figure 1.1B).

3. It is vital to leave leave the thermometer in position for the recommended length of time (usually 3 minutes). However, it does not affect accuracy if it is left for longer than the minimum time.

4. In accordance with the manufacturer's instructions, read the temperature by noting the way that the dots have changed colour (see Figure 1.1C).

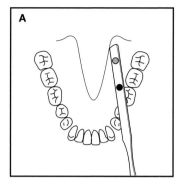

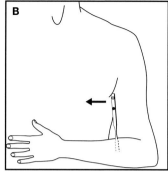

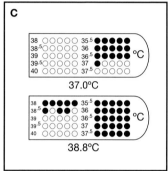

Figure 1.1 Disposable chemical thermometer. (A) Positioning the thermometer for oral use, (B) Positioning the thermometer for axillary use, (C) Reading the thermometer

Post procedure

Patient	Equipment/Environment	Nurse
• Ensure patient comfort.	• Dispose of the thermometer into the clinical waste bag.	• Record the temperature according to local policy. See page 16 for example of charting.
• Answer any questions regarding the recording.		• Report any abnormality. Normal range for adults 36°–37.2° Celcius.

Points for practice

1. If the patient is unconscious, confused, prone to seizures, has mouth sores or has undergone oral surgery, the oral site should not be used for temperature measurement. Temperature in the axilla is 0.5° lower than oral temperature. The rectal site is no longer recommended except when an electronic probe is being used.

2. Mercury thermometers are no longer widely used as there are risks of breakage. If a mercury thermometer is used, it must be cleaned before and after use and the mercury must be shaken down to the bottom of the scale before use.

3. Electronic oral and tympanic thermometers are increasingly being used (see page 5).

USE OF ELECTRONIC THERMOMETERS

Electronic thermometers are efficient, quick and easy to use, with an audible signal indicating that the reading is complete.

Oral and axilla

Oral

1. On the electronic machine select oral site.

2. Cover the probe with a disposable cover. Each cover is for use by one patient only and is usually kept clean and dry on the patient's locker between uses. It is discarded when the patient is discharged from the ward.

3. Place the covered probe under the tongue in the same way as a disposable thermometer (**Figure 1.2A**). When the audible signal is heard, remove the probe from the mouth. The temperature is shown in the digital display box.

Axilla

1. On the electronic machine select axilla site.

2. Cover the probe with a disposable cover. Each cover is for use by one patient only and is usually kept clean and dry on the patient's locker between uses. It is discarded when the patient is discharged from the ward.

3. Insert the probe horizontally and hold the arm close to the chest to ensure good contact with the skin. When the audible signal is heard, remove the probe from the axilla. The temperature is shown in the digital display box.

Tympanic

Tympanic thermometers are designed to measure the temperature by inserting a probe into the outer ear, adjacent to (but not touching) the tympanic membrane (**Figure 1.2B**). An infrared light detects heat radiated from the tympanic membrane and provides a digital reading. This usually takes only a few seconds and an audible signal indicates that the reading is complete. This provides a more accurate measurement of body core temperature as it is close to the carotid artery. A special cover is used for each patient to prevent cross-infection. It is a simple technique but the following may lead to an inaccurate reading: wax in the ear; a cracked or dirty lens; poor fitting in the ear; and if the patient has been recently lying on the ear that is used (Jevon 2001).

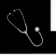

A

B

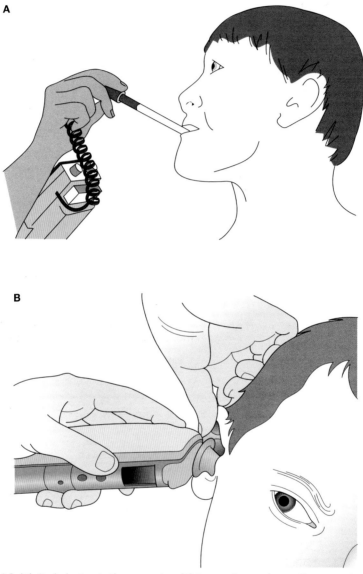

Figure 1.2 (A) Oral electronic thermometer, (B) tympanic membrane thermometer

COOLING THE PATIENT

Tepid sponging

Tepid sponging is designed to reduce the patient's temperature. The skin is cooled by applying tepid water with a sponge or flannel to a whole limb or extensive area of the body and then allowing it to evaporate, taking heat with it. With even a slightly raised temperature, this can make the patient feel much refreshed. It is important to maintain dignity and privacy throughout this procedure. Face cloths wrung out in tepid water and placed into the patient's axillae and groins will also assist cooling. Tepid rather than cold water is used, as cold water would cause peripheral vasoconstriction. Cold water might also induce shivering, which may cause the temperature to rise rather than fall. The temperature should be reduced by no more that 1°C per hour as cooling too rapidly can induce shock (Blows 2001).

Fan therapy

Cooling the air around the patient, so that the body loses more heat through radiation from the skin, is an effective way of cooling the person. However, it is important that the fan is carefully placed to avoid blowing onto the face of the patient as this can cause drying of the cornea of the eyes, leading to ulceration. The fan should be an oscillating type so that cooling is gentle and covers all areas of the body. As discussed above, cooling the skin too quickly may cause vasoconstriction, allowing less blood near the surface to be cooled.

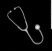

WARMING THE PATIENT

Patients, particularly the elderly, are often cold and may be suffering from hypothermia (a temperature of less than 35°C) on admission to hospital. This may be due to a lack of heating at home, exposure following an accident of some kind, or they may have been lying undiscovered for a period of time. It can also occur following lengthy surgery despite the use of warming methods during the operation. Warm air systems, which blow warm air through a disposable blanket onto the patient's body, are used to warm patients. A space blanket is made of thin, foil-type material that is designed to reflect back heat to prevent it being lost from the body. These are used in outdoor activities but are seen less often in the hospital setting. If the patient is receiving intravenous fluids or a blood transfusion, these can be warmed using a blood warmer (see page 106). If the patient is able to take oral fluids, hot drinks and soup are very effective. Humans lose a great deal of heat through their heads, so covering the head with a scarf or hat is beneficial. If the hypothermia is severe (temperature of less than 32°C), internal warming methods, such as warm gastric or peritoneal lavage and warmed intravenous fluids, may be necessary.

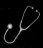
PULSE RECORDING

Preparation

Patient	Equipment/Environment	Nurse
• Explain the procedure, to gain consent and co-operation.	• A watch with a second hand.	• The hands should be clean. Additional protective clothing may be necessary if indicated by the patient's condition (see Chapter 9).
• The patient should be resting, either lying down or sitting. Allow at least 15 minutes rest after physical activity, emotional upset or smoking.	• Observation chart.	

Procedure

1. Choose a site to record the pulse. For most routine recordings the radial pulse is used (Figure 1.3) PFP1.

2. Using your first and second fingers to feel the pulse, lightly compress the artery PFP2.

3. Count the number of beats for 1 minute. If the pulse is regular, it is sufficient to count for 30 seconds and double the result. If the pulse is irregular, count for a full minute.

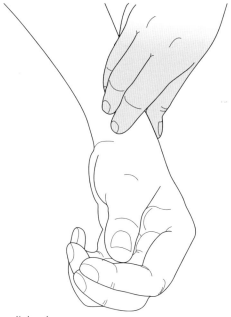

Figure 1.3 Taking the radial pulse

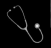
4. In addition to the rate per minute, note the rhythm, i.e. whether it is regular or irregular, and the volume/strength of the pulse felt **PFP3**.

5. Note the colour of the patient's skin and mucous membranes (inside lower eyelid). Pallor may indicate anaemia, while a bluish colour indicates a lack of oxygen (cyanosis, see page 12). In dark-skinned patients it is easier to detect this in the nail beds.

Post procedure

Patient

- Explain the results and discuss the reasons for any changes in care.

Nurse

- Record the findings according to local policy. See page 16 for an example of charting.

- Report any abnormalities **PFP4**.

Points for practice

1. The usual site for recording the pulse rate is at the wrist, where the radial pulse is easily felt. Pulses may also be felt at other sites (see page 28) and these may be used to check tissue perfusion (e.g. following surgery to a limb) or in an emergency when the radial pulse would not be appropriate.

2. Use light pressure only; pressing too hard can occlude the artery and you will not be able to feel the pulse. Do not use your thumb to feel the pulse. You have quite a strong pulse in your thumb and may feel your own pulse rather than the patient's.

3. It is important to feel the patient's pulse even if the pulse rate is shown on the pulse oximeter or automatic blood pressure machine. You need to feel the strength and the rhythm of the pulse.

4. The normal range in adults is 60–80 beats per minute.

ASSESSMENT OF BREATHING AND COUNTING RESPIRATIONS

Preparation

Patient	Equipment/Environment	Nurse
• The patient should be relaxed and resting, or recent activity should be noted. • Do not inform the patient when you will be assessing breathing **PFP1**.	• Watch with a second hand.	• The hands should be clean. • Additional protective clothing may be necessary if indicated by the patient's condition (see Chapter 9).

Procedure

1. Observe the movement of the chest wall for symmetry of chest movement and whether accessory muscles are being used **PFP2**.
2. Observe the rhythm and depth of respirations.
3. Count the respirations for 60 seconds **PFP3**.
4. Observe for the following:
   • Difficulty in breathing
   • Pain on breathing and its location
   • Noisy respiration – whether there is any wheeze or stridor
   • Cough – whether dry or productive
   • Sputum – amount, colour and consistency (see page 317).
5. Observe the patient's colour for signs of cyanosis **PFP4**.

Post procedure

Patient	Nurse
• Ensure the patient is comfortable. A patient with breathing difficulties may be most comfortable sitting upright (see page 302).	• Record/chart the respiratory observations according to local policy and report any abnormalities (see Figure 1.7 for an example of charting). • Adjust the frequency of observations as necessary.

Points for practice

1. A more accurate observation is obtained if the patient is unaware that their respirations are being counted. Many nurses achieve this by pretending to be feeling the radial pulse when in fact observing the movement of the chest wall (Figure 12.1 on page 301).

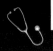

2. Accessory muscles are the sternocleidomastoid and trapezius muscles in the neck and shoulders. If these are being used it indicates that the patient is unable to use the diaphragm and external intercostal muscles adequately (Esmond 2001).

3. If breathing is very shallow and difficult to observe, lightly rest your hand on the patient's chest or abdomen to feel movement. The normal rate for an adult is 12–20 breaths per minute.

4. Cyanosis is a blue discoloration of the skin and mucous membranes and is most noticeable around the lips, earlobes, mouth and fingertips. In dark-skinned patients, signs of poor perfusion or cyanosis may be detected if the area around the lips or nail beds is dusky in colour.

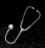

BLOOD PRESSURE RECORDING

Preparation

Patient	Equipment/Environment	Nurse
• Explain the procedure, to gain consent and co-operation.	• Sphygmomanometer with appropriate size cuff PFP2.	• The hands should be clean.
• The patient should be resting in a bed, couch or chair, in a quiet location, with their legs uncrossed.	• Stethoscope. • Alcohol-impregnated swabs.	• Additional protective clothing may be necessary if indicated by the patient's condition (see Chapter 9).
• The patient should not have had a meal, alcohol or caffeine or have smoked or exercised in the previous 30 minutes PFP1.	• Observation chart.	

Procedure

1. Assess the patient's knowledge of the procedure and explain as necessary.

2. Ensure the patient is resting in a comfortable position. If a comparison between lying and standing blood pressure is required, the 'lying' recording should be done first PFP1.

3. When applying the cuff, no clothing should be underneath it. If clothing constricts the arm, remove the arm from the sleeve PFP3.

4. Apply the cuff such that the centre of the 'bladder' is over the brachial artery, 2–3 cm above the antecubital fossa PFP4.

5. The arm should be positioned so that the cuff is level with the heart and may be more comfortable resting on a pillow PFP5.

6. The sphygmomanometer should be placed on a firm surface, with the dial clearly visible and the needle at zero.

7. Estimate systolic BP by locating the radial or brachial pulse. Squeeze the bulb slowly to inflate the cuff while still feeling the pulse. Observe the dial and note the level when the pulse can no longer be felt. Open the valve fully to quickly release the pressure in the cuff PFP6 (see Figure 1.4).

8. If using a communal stethoscope, clean the earpieces with an alcohol-impregnated swab. Curving the ends of the stethoscope slightly forward, place the earpieces in your ears. Check that the tubes are not twisted.

9. If the stethoscope has two sides, check that it is turned to the diaphragm side by tapping it with your finger (see Figure 1.5).

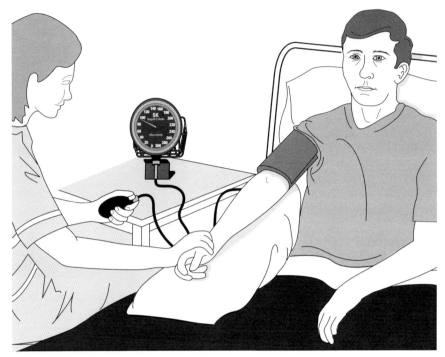

Figure 1.4 Estimating the systolic BP

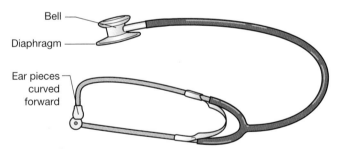

Figure 1.5 Stethoscope showing bell, diaphragm and earpieces

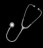
10. Palpate the brachial artery, which is located on the medial aspect of the antecubital fossa (just to the side of the midline, on the side nearest to the patient) (Figure 1.6).

11. Place the diaphragm of the stethoscope over the artery, and hold it in place with your thumb while your fingers support the patient's elbow (Figure 1.6) and ask the patient to relax their arm **PFP7**. You will not hear anything until the cuff is being deflated (step 14).

12. Position yourself so that the dial of the sphygmomanometer is clearly visible.

13. Ensure that the valve on the bulb is closed and inflate the cuff to 30 mmHg above the level noted in step 7. Open the valve to allow the needle of the dial to drop **slowly and steadily** (2 mm per second).

14. While observing the needle of the dial as it falls, listen for Korotkoff (thudding) sounds:
    - The **systolic** pressure is the level where these are first heard.
    - The **diastolic** pressure is the level where the sounds disappear.

15. Once the sounds have disappeared, open the valve fully, to completely deflate the cuff, and remove it from the patient's arm **PFP8**.

16. If a lying and standing BP is required, do not remove the cuff. Ask the patient to stand and then repeat steps 10–15 of the procedure **PFP9**.

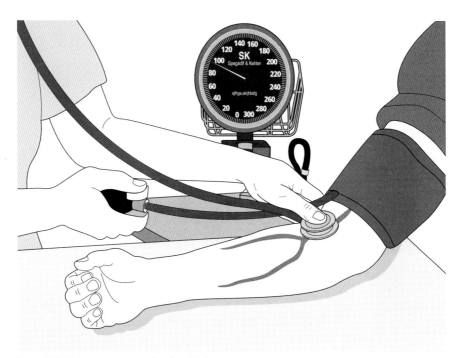

Figure 1.6 Stethoscope over the brachial artery

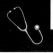

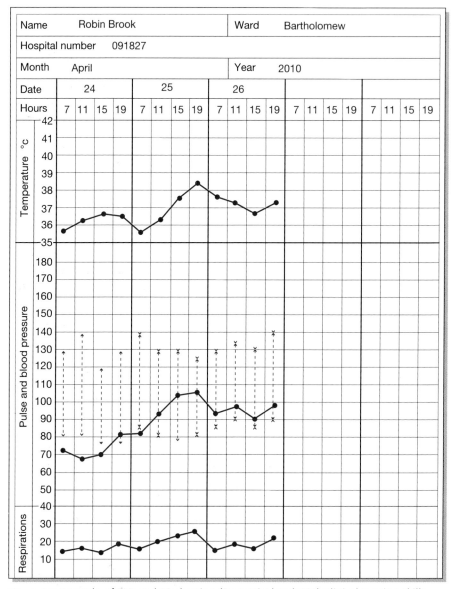

Figure 1.7 Example of TPR and BP charting (From Nicol M (2004) Clinical Nursing Skills Workbook. Mosby Elsevier).

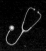

Post procedure

Patient	Equipment/Environment	Nurse
• Replace clothing and ensure the patient is comfortable.	• Replace equipment. • Clean the earpieces of the stethoscope.	• Record the blood pressure accurately according to local policy (see page 16 for example of charting). • Report any variation from previous recordings. The normal range in adults is 90/60 to 140/90.

Points for practice

1. The patient should be rested and lying or seated comfortably with the legs uncrossed and ideally should not have changed position for the previous 5 minutes. Where possible use the same arm for repeated BP measurements as it may vary 5–10 mmHg between arms (Blows 2001).

2. The sphygmomanometer may be an aneroid or a mercury type. These are used in exactly the same way except that a column of mercury, which must be placed in an upright position, is observed instead of a dial. Because mercury releases dangerous fumes if spilt, aneroid sphygmomanometers are replacing the mercury type. The bladder inside the cuff must cover at least 80% of the circumference of the upper arm (O'Brien et al 1997).

3. Electronic blood pressure recording machines are now commonly used. The cuff should be positioned in the same way as described in step 4, but no stethoscope is required because the machine provides a digital display of the systolic and diastolic pressures. These machines must be plugged into the mains electricity after use to re-charge the battery.

4. If the patient is receiving intravenous therapy, avoid using the arm that has the intravenous cannula or infusion in progress. Also avoid using the same arm as the pulse oximeter (see page 315).

5. The arm should be horizontal and supported at the level of the heart. If the arm is too low it could lead to over estimation of the systolic BP by up to 10 mmHg. If the arm is raised above the heart this may lead to under estimation (O'Brien et al 1997).

6. By estimating the systolic blood pressure in this way you avoid having to inflate the cuff unnecessarily high during step 13. Some authors (e.g. Blows 2001) suggest estimating the systolic BP by pumping the cuff up high and then feeling when the pulse returns, which we would argue may cause the patient unnecessary discomfort.

7. The arm should not be held rigid as muscle tension may cause a false reading (O'Brien et al 1997).

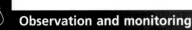

8. If you are unsure of the systolic or diastolic pressure you will need to re-inflate the cuff and repeat the procedure. If still unclear you should allow the patient to rest before repeating the procedure as repeated attempts may affect the accuracy of the reading.

9. If recording lying and standing blood pressure, do not remove the cuff between recordings, keep it in the same position. The doctor may have requested that the patient is standing for at least 5 minutes before the standing blood pressure is recorded. Be aware that the patient may feel dizzy on getting out of bed (postural hypotension).

CARDIAC MONITORING

Preparation

Patient	Equipment/Environment	Nurse
• Explain the procedure, to gain consent and co-operation. • Explain the need for bed rest while on the monitor **PFP1**. • Ensure privacy.	• Cardiac monitor with leads. This should have a maintenance sticker showing that it is safe to use. • Disposable electrodes. • Disposable razor or clippers (if required to remove body hair).	• The hands should be clean. • Additional protective clothing may be necessary if indicated by the patient's condition (see Chapter 9).

Procedure

1. Most acute areas will have wall-mounted cardiac monitors for use. If using a portable monitor, place it on a firm surface close to an electrical socket. Do not put anything on top of the monitor and keep the patient's drinks, etc., away from it.

2. Raise the bed to a safe working height (see Chapter 13 Moving and handling).

3. Expose the patient's chest and examine the sites that will be used for the electrodes.

4. If the chest is very hairy, shave a small patch at each site to allow good contact and adhesion of the electrodes.

5. Check the expiry date of the electrodes and ensure that they have not become dried out.

6. If the electrode has a small raised patch on the back, use this to roughen the skin slightly where the electrode will be placed. This improves adhesion and contact.

7. Remove the backing paper and taking care not to touch the gel in the middle, stick the electrodes firmly to the chest wall. The electrodes should be placed over bone and not muscle **PFP2**, avoiding areas that may be used for the placement of defibrillator pads.

8. Connect the leads to the electrodes. This is usually by means of a small clip or press stud. The leads are labelled or colour coded. If using a 3-lead system place the red electrode on the right shoulder, the yellow electrode on the left shoulder and the green electrode on the left lower abdomen (see Figure 1.8). If a 5-lead system is used, place the first three leads as detailed above, the black lead is placed on the lower right side of the abdomen and the white lead is placed in the middle of the chest **PFP3**.

9. Turn on the monitor and select lead II, which should produce the most positive (upright-looking) display. If lead II does not produce a good display, try lead I or lead III. If necessary, adjust the 'gain' on the monitor to make the display larger and easier to see.

10. Set the alarms to safe parameters, according to the patient's condition.

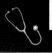

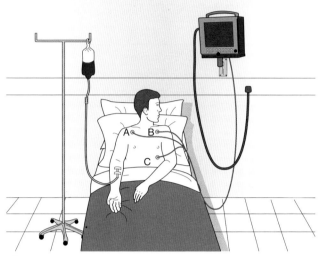

Figure 1.8 Cardiac monitoring

Post procedure

Patient	Equipment/Environment	Nurse
• Explain/demonstrate what will happen if the patient moves or disturbs the electrodes (i.e. abnormal-looking pattern) to prevent unnecessary concern. • Replace clothing and ensure that the leads are not pulling on the electrodes. • Lower the bed, adjusting the bed height for the patient's safety and convenience.	• Make sure all electrical cables are in good condition and are not under tension or trapped in any way, e.g. in back rest or bed rails. • Electrodes can usually remain in place for 24–72 hours, but may need replacing more frequently if the patient sweats a lot, if the electrode gel dries out, or if the patient's skin shows signs of sensitivity.	• Note the rhythm shown on the monitor and if the monitor has the facility, take a printout; it is a good idea to do this at the beginning of each shift. Put the patient's name, the date and time and sign the printout before filing in the notes. • Observe for any arrhythmias and report as appropriate.

Points for practice

1. In the acute situation, most patients with cardiac monitors are required to rest in bed. However, patients undergoing investigations for cardiac rhythm abnormalities may have a 24-hour tape (Holter monitor) or ambulatory monitoring system (telemetry), in which case they may move around, but should always inform the nurses of their whereabouts.

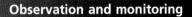

2. The electrodes should be placed over bone rather than muscle as muscle tremor will cause disruption on the ECG tracing.

3. The leads are referred to as limb leads even though they are attached to the chest. This is because they represent that area of the body, i.e. right arm, left arm and left leg.

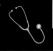
RECORDING A 12-LEAD ECG

Patient

- Explain the procedure, to gain consent and co-operation.
- Explain the need to lie still during the recording in order to gain a good trace.
- Ensure privacy.

Equipment/Environment

- A 12-lead electrocardiography (ECG) machine and leads, and paper for printout.
- Disposable electrodes for limb and chest leads (usually diposable, adhesive with clips or press studs).

Nurse

- The hands should be clean.
- Additional protective clothing may be necessary if indicated by the patient's condition (see Chapter 9).

Procedure

1. Ask/assist the patient to lie in a recumbent or semi-recumbent position.
2. Raise the bed to a safe working height (see Chapter 13 Moving and handling).
3. Expose the patient's ankles, wrists and chest area.
4. Apply the electrodes to the patient's ankles and wrists as shown in Figure 1.9A `PFP1`.
5. Apply the electrodes to the chest wall as described in Table 1.1 and shown in Figure 1.9B. If necessary, shave the area to ensure good contact/adhesion. In women with large or pendulous breasts it is sometimes difficult to place the chest leads under the breast. The electrodes may be placed over the breast in the appropriate position if this is the case.
6. Connect the ECG leads to the electrodes as labelled or colour coded.
7. Ask the patient to lie still during the recording to avoid artefact being recorded on the trace.
8. Press 'start' on the ECG machine. All 12 leads (views of the heart) will print out on one page. Add the patient's name, ward and hospital number to the printout `PFP2`.

Table 1.1 Chest lead positions for 12-lead ECG

V1	Right sternal border, 4th intercostal space
V2	Left sternal border, 4th intercostal space
V3	Located directly between V2 and V4 (place V4 prior to V3)
V4	5th intercostal space, mid-clavicular line
V5	5th intercostal space, anterior axillary line
V6	Same plane as V4 and V5, mid axillary line

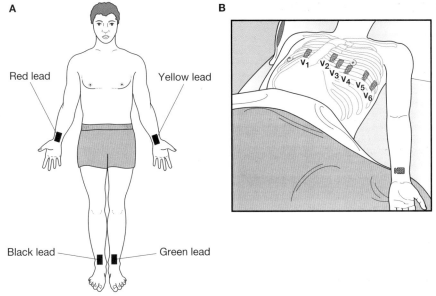

Figure 1.9 (A) 12-lead ECG position of limb leads, (B) position of chest leads

Post procedure

Patient	Equipment/Environment	Nurse
• Remove the electrodes and wipe away any traces of gel.	• Leave the ECG machine clean, tidy and stocked ready for the next user. Do not tie the leads together as this may damage them.	• File the ECG printout in the patient's notes.
• Help the patient to replace clothing.		• Inform the requesting practitioner that the ECG is available.
• Lower the bed to a safe level.		
• Ensure the patient is comfortable.		

Points for practice

1. If the patient is an amputee, apply the electrode to the stump.
2. It is usual to note whether the patient has chest pain or is pain free at the time of the ECG recording. In some hospitals it is policy for the person recording the ECG to date and sign the printout.

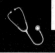

OBSERVATION OF LIMB PERFUSION, MOVEMENT AND SENSATION

Preparation

Patient	Equipment/Environment	Nurse
• Explain procedure, to gain consent and co-operation. • Explain the need for frequent observations **PFP1**.	• Screening the bed is not usually necessary, but ensure that dignity and privacy are maintained.	• Hands must be clean. • Additional protective clothing may be necessary if indicated by the patient's condition (see Chapter 9).

Procedure

Assess the following **PFP2**:

1. Movement – ask the patient to move the toes/fingers of the affected area of the limb.

2. Sensation – without letting the patient see which toes/fingers you are touching, touch the toes/fingers randomly and ask the patient to tell you which one you are touching **PFP3**.

3. Perfusion – in order to assess perfusion observe the following:
   • temperature – the fingers/toes should be warm to touch
   • colour – the skin should be pink, indicating adequate perfusion. If the patient has dark skin, observe the nail beds
   • pulse – it may not always be possible to locate a pulse, particularly in the feet. Therefore, once located (Figure 1.10), it is helpful to mark the site to make it easier for subsequent checking. If bandages or a splint prevent you locating a pulse this should be documented **PFP4**.

4. Pain/swelling – if the patient complains of pain or the toes/fingers are swollen, check the bandage, splint or plaster cast for tightness.

5. Bandage/dressing/splint/plaster cast – check for bleeding and that the bandage/dressing/splint is not too tight, causing constriction of the blood supply to the limb.

Post procedure

Patient	Equipment/Environment	Nurse
• Elevation of the affected limb will help prevent swelling. • The elevated limb must be well supported.	• Exposed extremities may be kept warm by using a loose-fitting sock or piece of tubular bandage.	• Wash hands. • Document findings according to local policy; these are usually incorporated into the main observation chart.

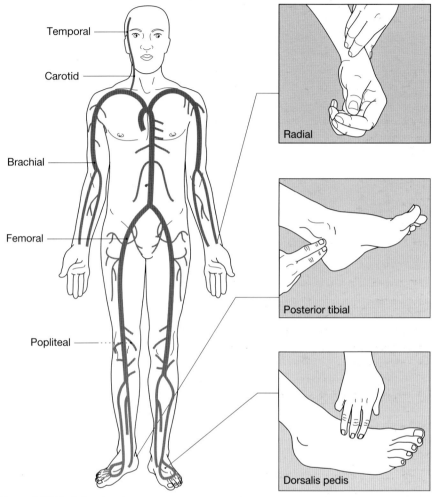

Figure 1.10 Peripheral pulses

Points for practice

1. These observations are made following injury or surgery to a limb. The limb may be bandaged, splinted or encased in plaster of Paris.

2. When observing limb perfusion, movement and sensation it is often helpful to compare it to the other limb, if that is unaffected.

3. It is important to see all the fingers/toes move, particularly as little toes can be covered. Each digit has a separate nerve supply, which may be damaged or compressed.

4. If recording 'pulse not felt', take care that it is not confused with 'pulse not able to be located' due to the bandage/splint, etc.

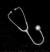

ASSESSMENT OF LEVEL OF CONSCIOUSNESS

Preparation

Patient

- Explain the need for frequent observations, even throughout the night. Observations must be continued and sleeping patients must be woken to check that they are not in a coma.

Equipment/Environment

- A small, bright torch for pupil reactions.
- Sphygmomanometer, stethoscope and thermometer.
- Neurological assessment chart (see page 30).
- If the patient is confused and restless, bed rails padded with pillows may be needed. The bed should be at its lowest level.

Nurse

- The hands should be clean.
- Additional protective clothing may be necessary if indicated by the patient's condition (see Chapter 9).

Procedure

The Glasgow Coma Scale (page 31) was developed to assess the depth of impaired consciousness using an objective tool whose purpose is to avoid inconsistency when using different assessors (Palmer & Knight 2006). Level of consciousness is determined by monitoring the patient's ability in eye opening, motor response and verbal response. Each activity is scored independently according to the stimulus needed to elicit a response from the patient. The worst total score is 3 and the best 15. Any reduction in the score is a sign that the patient's consciousness level is deteriorating and should be reported immediately. A patient with a score of 8 or less will be in a deep coma. Three levels of stimuli are usually adopted: auditory (a question, a command or a noise, like hand clapping); tactile (touch); and painful stimuli, which are considered the most powerful.

Assessment of eye opening

Eye opening demonstrates that the arousal mechanisms in the brain are functioning and the scoring system is used as follows:

4 = patients who are conscious, who sense your approach and open their eyes spontaneously or patients who are asleep, but open their eyes in response to a verbal stimulus or light touch.

3 = patients who open their eyes in response to a verbal stimulus.

2 = patients who open their eyes only in response to a painful stimulus.
   The normal response to pain is to draw away from the stimulus by moving the limb or trying to push the nurse's hand away. There is much debate in the literature in respect of the use of painful stimuli (Price 2002, Palmer & Knight 2006). These are either peripheral stimuli (pressing firmly on the side

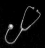
of the finger or the earlobe) or central stimuli by trapezium squeeze (pinching and twisting the muscle where the head meets the shoulder) or supra-orbital pressure (firm pressure in the eye socket just above the eye). The consensus appears to be that pain response is best assessed centrally as a response is an indicator that the motor pathways are still functioning to some extent (McLeod 2004). Peripheral stimuli, although useful when assessing an individual limb that has not moved in response to a central stimulus, could also be a reflex activity. Other methods (e.g. rubbing the sternum with the knuckles or pressing on nail beds) are not recommended.

1 = no eye opening in response to verbal or painful stimuli. Patients may not be able to open their eyes if there is damage to the oculomotor nerve, which is responsible for movement of the eyelid. If the patient is unable to open their eyes due to swelling, trauma or an eye dressing, this is indicated using the letter 'C'. If unable to open their eyes due to medication (e.g. paralysing agents) this is indicated using the letter 'P'.

Verbal response

This assesses whether patients are aware of themselves and their environment. If the patient has a tracheostomy or an endotracheal tube, the letter 'T' can be used to indicate this. The score is used as follows:

5 = the patient is orientated, i.e. able to tell the nurse who they are, where they are, what day, date, month and year it is, and why they are where they are.

4 = the patient is able to hold a conversation, but not able to answer specific questions (i.e. confused and not orientated).

3 = the patient can speak, but does so randomly and makes verbal responses such as swearing or shouting.

2 = speech is incomprehensible and the nurse may have to use painful stimuli to get a response.

1 = the patient does not respond to verbal and painful stimuli.

If the patient is unable to speak (dysphasia) it may be due to damage to speech centres in the brain. There are two types: receptive dysphasia (when patients cannot understand the spoken word) and expressive dysphasia (when they are unable to reply with the correct words). In both cases, a score of 1 is given and the dysphasia is noted by using the letter 'D'.

Motor response

When assessing motor response, scores are allocated as follows:

6 = obeying commands (the best response). Instructions may include 'lift your arms' or 'squeeze my hands'.

5 = localising to pain, which means that the patient's brain is receiving sensory information regarding the process of feeling pain. When assessing for this response a central pain stimulus (see 'Assessment of eye opening' above) is used. Patients will usually respond by trying purposefully to remove the source of the pain. An arm is used to test this because leg responses are less reliable and can be a spinal reflex rather than a brain response. If the patient cannot be assessed due to presence of fractures, this can be documented using the symbol '#'. The best (and safest) stimulus to assess this response is the trapezium squeeze (see 'Assessment of eye opening' above).

4 = the patient withdraws from pain or moves towards the source of the pain, but does not attempt to remove it.

3 = abnormal flexion, which is an abnormal response such as wrist rotation and arm or elbow flexion. This usually indicates that the nerve pathways are not functioning normally and in some cases is a sign of deterioration and a poor prognosis.

2 = the patient extends to pain and may rotate the arm inwards or extend or straighten the arm at the elbow. This indicates damage to the brain stem and the prognosis for the patient is very poor.

1 = no response to pain. Patients who are deemed to be 'brain dead' will score 1.

Pupil response

Raised intracranial pressure causes changes in the size of the pupils and their response to light. Assessment of the pupils (Figure 1.11) assesses the function of the optic nerve, which causes a reaction to light being shone in the eye, and the oculomotor nerve, which constricts the pupil. A poor reaction in either of these assessments indicates compression of the nerves. When undertaking assessment

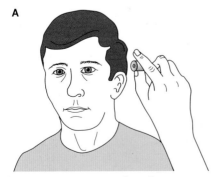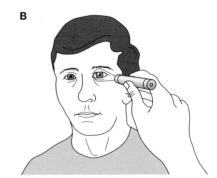

Figure 1.11 Assessment of pupil response

of the pupils, dim the light in the room and hold the eyelid open. Before you shine the light in the patient's eye observe the following:

- The resting size of both pupils. The average size is 2–5 mm, but it varies according to the time of the day
- Whether both pupils are equal in size – inequality can be a serious sign of raised intracranial pressure
- The shape of the pupils – they are normally round. Different shapes can indicate damage to the brain.

Bringing the light of the pen torch in from the side of the eye, observe:

- the reaction of each pupil to light
- the intensity of the reaction, i.e. whether it is brisk, sluggish or absent.

It is also important to note if the patient has a pre-existing abnormality or irregularity of the eye/s, for example cataracts, which will affect the response. In addition it is important to note any drugs or medications the patients may have had. Some cause dilation (e.g. atropine) whilst others (opiates, e.g. morphine) cause constriction.

Vital signs

These are not part of the Glasgow Coma Scale itself but because of their importance, they are usually included on the same chart (Figure 1.12):

- **Temperature** – alterations in patients' temperature may be due to damage of the thermoregulation centre of the brain. A rise in body temperature increases the demand for oxygen by the brain cells, which may already be compromised due to damage. It is desirable to keep the body temperature within normal limits, where possible. This may require antipyretic agents such as paracetamol or active measures such as fan therapy (see page 7).
- **Pulse rate and blood pressure** – in patients with raised intracranial pressure the blood pressure rises and pulse rate falls. As the brain becomes hypoxic and ischaemic, the body responds by attempting to increase the arterial blood pressure in order to get oxygen to it. As a result there is a need for more blood in each contraction of the heart. This results in a slowing of the heart rate (bradycardia). Respiration rate also decreases and a change in the respiratory pattern occurs (see below). This is known as 'Cushing's reflex' and is a very late occurrence after level of consciousness deteriorates. Careful recording and charting is needed so that a trend in this direction is clearly detectable.
- **Respiration rate** – changes in respiration are a good indicator of the function of the brain stem. This is because there are four respiratory control centres in two parts of the brain stem. Monitoring of respiration rate and pattern is essential as a sudden change, such as Cheyne–Stokes breathing (deep, sighing respirations followed by periods of apnoea for several seconds) or apnoea, is due to a significant rise in intracranial pressure.

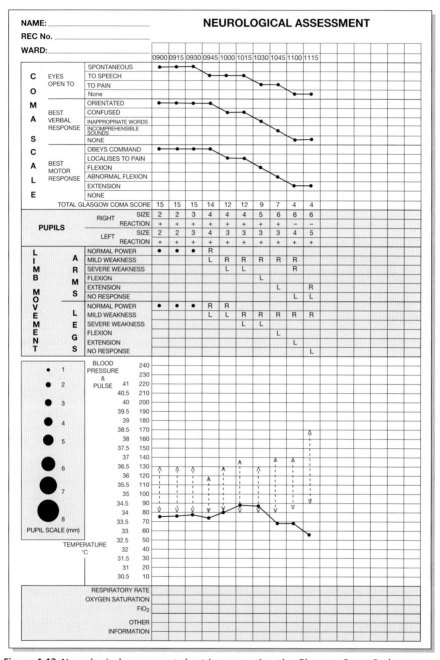

Figure 1.12 Neurological assessment chart incorporating the Glasgow Coma Scale

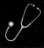

Limb movement

In addition to motor response assessment, assessing limb movement can detect weaknesses of one side of the body or limbs. Assessing limb movement and motor power gives an indication of the extent of the damage to the motor cortex that controls motor movement and is graded as follows:

- **Normal power** – the nurse applies resistance to any joint movement and this can be matched by the patient, e.g. pulling or pushing whilst holding the hands.
- **Mild weakness** – the patient is able to counter the resistance, but is easily overcome.
- **Severe weakness** – the patient is able to move the limb but not against resistance.
- **Flexion, extension or no response** – there is flexion, extension or no movement in response to central or peripheral painful stimuli.

Other level of consciousness assessment tools

In recent years alternative assessment tools, such as the AVPU (alert, responds to voice, pain or unresponsive) have emerged. The AVPU has a simple structure, which is easy to apply and has been incorporated into the Early Warning Score (EWS, also known as Patient At Risk (PAR) score) (Palmer & Knight 2006). This is in recognition of the fact that many patients who are critically ill will have altered levels of consciousness. The AVPU can give information quickly about a patient's level of consciousness, which can be more formally assessed with the Glasgow Coma Scale as necessary. However, it should not replace the Glasgow Coma Scale as an assessment tool (McLeod 2004).

CARE OF THE PATIENT HAVING A SEIZURE

Preparation

Patient	Equipment/Environment	Nurse
• Protecting the patient from injury is of primary concern. • Maintain privacy and dignity where possible PFP1.	• Ensure patient safety. This may entail clearing the environment or, on rare occasions, moving the patient from danger.	• Maintain own safety. • Protective clothing may be necessary if indicated by the patient's condition (see Chapter 9).

Procedure

When the patient has a seizure PFP2, the first phase (the tonic phase) is associated with rigidity of limbs and breath holding. This phase may be brief. In the second phase (clonic phase), there is rhythmical jerking of arms and legs. Characteristically the jerks are unilateral; initially close together and then decreasing in frequency. This phase is followed by a period of deep sleep, when the patient is usually unrousable and their body is limp:

1. Protect the patient from injury, but do not attempt to restrain their limbs.

2. Use pillows as necessary to pad hard surfaces, and remove non-essential furniture and equipment.

3. Observe the patient continuously, noting the following:
   - duration of each phase of the seizure, including the recovery time (i.e. when able to resume normal activities)
   - limbs involved
   - whether movement is localised or general
   - whether the jaw is clenched PFP3
   - whether the patient is frothing at the mouth (saliva)
   - whether the patient has been incontinent of urine or faeces
   - breathing pattern – this will change. Patients are likely to hold their breath and may become cyanosed or just pale. Loud breathing sounds may indicate the end of the seizure. (The breathing reverts spontaneously and oxygen is not usually required.)

4. During the period of deep sleep following the clonic phase, the patient should be left in the recovery position to maintain an airway and should not be disturbed, allowing the patient to recover in their own time. It can last up to 30 minutes.

5. It is now safe to put your fingers in the patient's mouth to remove food or dentures if necessary.

6. If a seizure or seizures occur in rapid succession and last 30 minutes or longer this is called *status epilepticus* (Walker 2005). This requires urgent medical intervention.

Post procedure

Patient	Equipment/Environment	Nurse
• Reassure patient by being calm and explaining what has happened.	• Ensure patient comfort by offering a wash, change of clothing, etc., as necessary.	• All seizures must be documented and reported.
• Ask patient whether there was any warning of the seizure (aura) and whether it can be described, e.g. a smell or taste.		• If there is no previous history of seizures or a change in the pattern/length of seizures, the doctor should be informed.

Points for practice

1. If the seizure occurs in a public place, encourage bystanders to disperse to prevent the patient feeling crowded and possibly embarrassed.

2. The term seizure was previously referred to as 'fitting'. A seizure with tonic and clonic phases was formerly called a grand mal fit.

3. During the tonic phase of the seizure, the patient will clench their jaw and may bite their tongue. Nothing should be inserted into the mouth to try and prevent this.

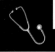
WEIGHING PATIENTS

Preparation

Patient	Equipment/Environment	Nurse
• Encourage the patient to empty their bladder.	• The scales must be on a level surface.	• The hands should be clean.
• Weigh the patient on the same scales, at the same time each day/week, and in similar clothing **PFP1**.	• Use the same scales for regular weighing **PFP1**. • Ensure the pointer is at zero or weights are to the left, at zero.	• An apron should be worn if the patient requires assistance. Additional protective clothing may be necessary if indicated by the patient's condition (see Chapter 9).

Procedure

1. Position the scales for easy access and apply the brakes.
2. Ask/assist the patient to sit on the scales or stand on the platform. If electronic scales are being used, plug them in to the mains before the patient sits down.
3. If sitting, ensure that the patient's feet are off the floor (Figure 1.13).

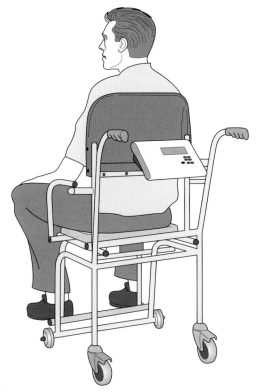

Figure 1.13 Weighing a patient

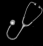

4. Ask the patient to remain still and note the reading.

5. If the scales are electric the weight will be displayed. If manual scales are used check the patient's previous weight to determine the approximate position and move the heavier weight bar (kilograms) to the right until the two pivotal arrows swing (e.g. if the previous weight was 73 kg, move the heavier bar to 70 kg). If the bar is moved too far, the weight will sink and stop swinging. Adjust the lighter weight bar so that the arrows are exactly level and free floating.

6. Note the reading by adding the position of the heavier bar (e.g. 70 kg) to that of the lighter bar (e.g. 3.5 kg; total equals 73.5 kg).

7. If the weight is very different from a recent previous weight, check it again and, if confirmed, report it.

Post procedure

Patient	Equipment/Environment	Nurse
• Assist the patient back to the bed/chair as necessary.	• Return the scales to their storage place and clean if necessary.	• Document weight and report any unexpected loss or gain.

Points for practice

1. It is important to use the same set of scales for regular weighing as there will be variation between sets of scales. The actual weight is usually of less importance than whether the weight is increasing or decreasing; it will not be possible to accurately detect changes unless the same scales are used and the patient is wearing similar clothing at the same time of day.

BLOOD GLUCOSE MONITORING

Preparation

Patient	Equipment/Environment	Nurse
• Explain the procedure, to gain consent and co-operation.	• Blood glucose meter.	• Most Trusts require nurses to have undergone formal training in the use of the glucometer – check local policy.
• Ensure the patient's hands are clean. Do not use alcohol wipes **PFP1**.	• Finger-pricking device or lancet.	
	• Gauze swab/cotton-wool ball, according to local policy.	• The hands should be clean and apron and gloves should be worn.
• Ask the patient to choose the finger to be used for the procedure.	• Blood glucose testing strips.	• Additional protective clothing may be necessary if indicated by the patient's condition (see Chapter 9).

Procedure

1. Ensure all equipment is within easy reach and the patient is comfortable.
2. If necessary, assist the patient with washing and drying of the finger/hand.
3. Use new lancets and platforms (if finger-pricking device used) for each test **PFP2**.
4. Check the expiry date of the testing strips and prepare the blood glucose meter and insert the testing strip according to the manufacturer's instructions **PFP3**.
5. Using the appropriate device, prick the side of the patient's fingertip. Avoid frequent use of the thumbs, index and little fingers where possible **PFP4**.
6. Allow a drop of blood to fall onto the testing strip – do not smear **PFP5**.
7. Ask the patient to press on the site, using the gauze swab/cotton-wool ball, to stem bleeding and reduce the risk of bruising.
8. Wait for the meter to provide a digital display of the result **PFP6**.

Post procedure

Patient	Equipment/Environment	Nurse
• Ensure the patient is comfortable.	• Dispose of all sharps and contaminated waste in the appropriate containers.	• Remove gloves and wash hands.
• Inform the patient of their blood glucose level.	• Return equipment as appropriate.	• Document the result and report any abnormalities.
• Ensure bleeding has stopped.		

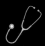

Points for practice

1. The patient's hands should be clean and washing the hands in warm water will encourage blood flow. If the patient is unable to wash their hands, and there is any possibility that there may have been contact with substances such as fruit juice, the finger should be washed or wiped with a wet tissue and then a dry tissue before pricking (Walker 2004). An alcohol swab must not be used as this may give a false reading (Burden 2001).

2. Where possible use a finger-pricking device, as it is more likely to ensure a good blood flow and is less painful (Burden 2001). Before pricking the patient's finger, hold the hand downwards to encourage blood flow, and make a light tourniquet with your hand around the finger to ensure sufficient blood is present in the tip of the finger. Avoid 'milking' blood into the finger as the local blood composition may be disturbed by intermingling with tissue fluid. Taking time to encourage blood flow before pricking the finger will reduce the need for pricking again, which can be distressing for the patient.

3. Preparation of the glucose meter usually involves checking that it has been calibrated for the particular batch of testing strips that are being used.

4. The side of the patient's finger is used as it is less painful. However, the site should be rotated because even using the side of the finger can be painful, especially if performed several times a day (Walker 2004). This also helps reduce the risk of infection from multiple finger pricks and prevents the area from becoming hardened.

5. The drop of blood should fall onto the strip rather than be 'wiped on', as this may lead to an inaccurate result. Test strips do vary and with some the blood is not dropped directly onto the strip. Always check the manufacturer's instructions.

6. With some glucose meters, the strip is inserted into the monitor after the blood is dropped onto it. Follow the manufacturer's instructions regarding timing and wiping prior to insertion into the machine.

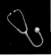

PAIN ASSESSMENT

Principles

Pain is sometimes considered to be the fifth vital sign (after temperature, pulse, respirations and BP), which indicates the level of importance that should be placed on assessing and managing pain (Lynch 2001). This is because pain can have harmful physiological, psychological and emotional effects. Pain is a complex phenomenon and its successful management has always presented a challenge. There have been significant advances in the management of pain with the development of acute and chronic pain services, and improved techniques for administering analgesia, including patient-controlled analgesia (PCA) and epidural analgesia. There is also a greater recognition of the role of non-pharmacological strategies in the management of pain. Effective pain management depends on good interprofessional team working, and the nurse's role is central in ensuring that the patient's pain is assessed, treatment regimens are implemented and their effectiveness evaluated. Successful pain management depends on accurate assessment and reassessment of the patient's pain (Davies & McVicar 2000a). Given its complexity not only must the sensory component be assessed but also the patient's moods, attitudes, coping efforts, resources and its impact on their lives and those of their family. This is a continuous process and it is suggested here that there are three key areas for consideration in the assessment of pain. The extent of the assessment will vary with specific circumstances.

1. Who should assess the patient's pain?

Pain is largely a subjective experience and so patients themselves are best placed to assess their own pain accurately (McCaffery & Ferrell 1997). Observation by others involves interpretation of what the patient is feeling and, therefore, can be unreliable. It is vital that nurses accept the patients' estimation of their pain even if it is not accompanied by the usual behaviours (e.g. grimacing, adopting a foetal position, groaning) or alteration to vital signs, e.g. raised pulse. Vital signs can be unreliable as a measure of a person's pain. The way in which different patients respond to pain can be attributed to a multitude of variables, such as age, culture, type of pain and duration. Observation and vital-sign measurement should only be relied upon when the patient is unable to communicate. Assessment of pain is an important aspect of the nurse's role that requires a number of skills, including observation, interpretation and communication skills.

2. When should the patient's pain be assessed?

The frequency of pain assessment is dependent on the individual circumstances. Factors to be considered when determining frequency include:

- The severity of the pain. Pain assessment is often carried out when the patient is resting, but a better indicator of the efficacy of analgesia will be achieved by asking the patient to cough, move or take a deep breath.
- Frequency of assessment should be increased if pain is poorly controlled or treatment regimens are changing.

- Regular pain assessment is important in the post-operative period. Patients with patient-controlled analgesia (PCA – see page 42) should be assessed each time other vital signs are recorded. In patients with epidural analgesia (see page 45), the sensory block should be checked approximately 20 minutes after the administration of the analgesic.

3. What should be assessed?

Multidimensional pain tools such as the McGill Pain Questionnaire (MPQ) offer a framework for assessment of many of the issues outlined below and include the intensity, sensory, affective and evaluative elements of pain. However, no one tool is adequate for enabling the patient to describe the quality of their pain experience and what is more important is facilitating the telling of their 'story' through open questions, active listening and reflecting (Davies & McVicar 2000).

Initial assessment of a patient's pain should include:

- **The location, duration, intensity and characteristics of the pain**
  Defining the nature of a patient's pain is important, as different types of pain will be treated differently. The nurse should establish whether the pain is localised to a particular part of the body or whether it is more generalised. The patient should be asked to describe whether the pain is 'sharp', 'dull', 'intermittent' or 'continuous', and to indicate when did it start and how long they have had it. The patient's perception of the pain is important and this should be assessed in terms of whether it is 'tolerable', 'unbearable', etc.

- **The underlying condition**
  The underlying diagnosis or cause of a patient's pain is central to determining whether the subsequent treatment is curative or palliative. For example, acute pain is often an indicator of disease or injury, which following treatment can be resolved. Conversely, pain may indicate a worsening of the patient's condition, but the overall goal of treatment may be palliative and focus on relieving the symptoms.

- **Is the pain acute, persistent (chronic) or referred?**
  It is important to establish whether the patient's pain is acute, persistent (chronic) or referred, as this may influence the choice of treatment. For example, pharmacological intervention is the mainstay of acute pain management, whereas chronic pain management often demands a range of treatment options including pharmacological and non-pharmacological regimens. Chronic pain is increasingly being referred to as persistent pain, with some distinguishing between that which is caused by tissue damage (nociceptive) or that which has persisted beyond the original cause as a result of disruption to the normal transmission of pain (neuropathic) (Duke 2006). This important physiological distinction has the advantage of informing decision-making about the best way to manage the pain. Referred pain is common in conditions that originate in the viscera. For example, the pain in a myocardial infarction is often referred to the left arm.

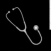

- **Any medical/nursing treatment being given**
  Any treatment currently being received by the patient should be
  reviewed in order to determine its effectiveness. Furthermore, current
  treatment may be an important indicator as to the efficacy of any proposed
  treatments.

- **Precipitating or exacerbating factors, e.g. mobility/immobility, time of day, eating/drinking**
  Determining factors that precipitate or exacerbate the pain facilitates diagnosis
  and also aids with identification of the goals of care. For example, if a patient
  develops pain when undertaking a particular activity, the goal of care may be
  twofold. The patient may be encouraged to either avoid the activity or may
  undertake a programme that concentrates on maximising their coping
  potential in that situation. Time of day may also be significant; some patients
  report higher levels of pain at night.

- **Related symptoms, e.g. nausea, vomiting, breathlessness or sleeplessness**
  Related symptoms, such as nausea and vomiting, are often significant in
  aiding diagnosis, but are also important in that they can cause the patient such
  distress as to interfere with their ability to cope with pain. A score to indicate
  the level of nausea and vomiting is often used with patients receiving PCA.
  This should be assessed and recorded with other vital signs. Pain that causes
  sleeplessness significantly reduces the patient's ability to tolerate it.

- **Coping strategies used by the patient – pharmacological and non-pharmacological**
  When determining the plan of care for a patient in pain, it is important to
  include any coping strategies the patient may have developed. Medication
  used by the patient may indicate what 'works' and may subsequently minimise
  the risk of prescribing treatments that 'do not work'. Non-pharmacological
  coping strategies (such as use of heat pads or massage) should, whenever
  possible, be included in the overall plan of care. This will enhance the patient's
  perception of being involved in their plan of care.

- **Meaning or significance of the pain for the patient**
  The patient's perception of the significance of their pain is extremely
  important. Pain creates fear, anxiety and a sense of loss of control. Fear of
  death is common. It is essential, therefore, for the nurse to establish how
  patients perceive their pain.

Self-report pain assessment tools

It is vital that nurses regard pain assessment as a priority. Unless pain is assessed
regularly and effectively, patients will continue to suffer unnecessarily. Effective
pain assessment is a fundamental part of nursing care and accountability for the
accuracy of pain assessment lies firmly within the domain of nursing. However,
because of the subjective nature of the pain experience, feedback from patients
about the intensity of their pain experiences is essential. Initial and ongoing assessment may be undertaken using a Self-Reporting Pain Assessment Tool, but it is

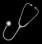

important to remember that they only rate pain intensity, which is only one aspect of the patient's pain experience. The most commonly used are:

- **Visual Analogue Scale**
  The Visual Analogue Scale uses a 10-cm line with one end-point indicating 'No Pain' and the other indicating 'Worst Pain Imaginable' (Figure 1.14). The patient indicates the point on the line that best represents their pain. Some scales include words at set intervals, e.g. 'slight', 'moderate', 'severe'.

- **Verbal Numerical Rating Scale**
  The Verbal Numerical Rating Scale is similar to the Visual Analogue Scale. Using a scale in which 0 is 'no pain' and 10 is 'worst imaginable pain', patients are asked to indicate the number that best represents their pain.

- **Verbal Rating Scale**
  These scales ask the patient to consider a series of words that best describes the pain, e.g. 'none', 'mild', 'moderate', 'severe', 'very severe' and 'worst pain imaginable'.

Any of the above scales may be complemented by the use of a body outline that gives a good indication of pain sites. Providing the patient is able to understand the tool there are a number of advantages to using such scales:

- They can be used alone or in conjunction with other pain assessment.
- They are simple to use.
- They provide a clear picture of pain intensity.
- Regular use provides evidence of the efficacy of treatment regimens and indicates an improvement or worsening of the patient's pain experience.

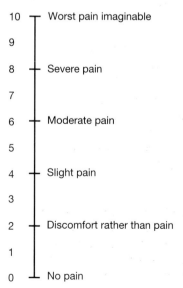

Figure 1.14 Visual Analogue Scale

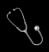

PATIENT-CONTROLLED ANALGESIA (PCA)

Principles

Patient-controlled analgesia (PCA) has become a popular method of managing post-operative pain since the early 1990s. However, today its use is not confined to post-operative pain management; it has been found to be useful in patients with burns, myocardial infarction, bone marrow transplantation and sickle cell crisis. It can also be useful with patients who are terminally ill. PCA facilitates active involvement of patients in the management of their pain. Through the use of a syringe driver and a timing device, PCA allows patients to self-administer small doses of an analgesic whenever they feel pain. It has several advantages over intermittent intramuscular or subcutaneous administration of analgesics on an 'as required' basis:

1. PCA gives the patient a sense of control and there is no questioning of the validity of the pain.
2. It enables analgesia requirement to be individualised to a sufficiently high plasma concentration level and stable plasma concentration levels to be maintained thereafter. This prevents the peaks and troughs associated with intermittent injection.
3. Unlike the conventional system of intermittent injection, there is no delay between the request for analgesia and the provision of pain relief.
4. It saves nurses' time.

PCA is usually administered intravenously (although epidural and subcutaneous infusions are also possible) via a syringe driver and timing device. The patient activates the system by pressing a button that releases a small dose of the analgesic into the circulation. There is a 'lock-out' device that prevents further doses being delivered with a specified time interval (usually between 5 and 20 minutes depending on the drug and the dosage). The use of the lock-out device reduces the risk of overdose. Morphine is the most common opiate used and a dose of 1 mg at 10-minute intervals will usually provide effective pain relief with minimal side effects, provided the patient is carefully monitored throughout (see below).

PCA devices

There is a variety of battery or electrically operated PCA devices available. Most will include the following features:

- A lock-out device that prevents the syringe driver delivering more than the maximum preset dose over a set period, e.g. 4 hours
- Safety features that include alarms for occlusion (blockage), air in the line, low battery or empty syringe
- A keypad lock and other locking devices that prevent unauthorised access and changes to the programme
- An electronic microprocessor that allows the flow rate, bolus dose and lock-out interval to be set. This will usually record the number of bolus doses

requested and administered, which is important when determining the effectiveness of the PCA

• Anti-syphon valves and anti-reflux valves should be used.

An alternative is a mechanical system where a 'control module' is worn around the wrist with a connecting pocket-sized infusor. This is less flexible than the electronic pumps as it only delivers a pre-set, non-adjustable volume and has only one lock-out interval and no safety alarms. However, it is much cheaper than the electronic modes and affords the patient greater freedom of movement.

Patient education

The successful use of PCA is dependent on the patient being willing and able to use it. Therefore, patient education is vital, and with surgical patients this should occur pre-operatively, either in the pre-admission clinic or on the ward. The patient should be encouraged to handle the device and press the buttons, etc., in order to become familiar with the device to be used. It is important that the nurse notes the patient's understanding and dexterity in handling the equipment because patients who are unable to manage the device may not receive any analgesia. If a patient is unable to use the system, nurse-administered analgesia will be required.

Monitoring the patient

Regular monitoring is essential for patients with a PCA. This includes the following:

1. Ensuring the machine is placed at or below the level of the patient's heart to prevent any risk of siphoning.

2. Close monitoring of respiration rate, particularly immediately after commencement, as respiratory depression is the main side effect of opiate analgesia. Local protocol should be consulted regarding the action to be taken if respirations fall below a certain level; a respiratory rate of less than 8 or 10 respirations a minute usually requires intervention from the pain control nurse, the anaesthetist or doctor. Some protocols stipulate that patients should have oxygen administered whilst the PCA is in progress. Oxygen saturation levels should be recorded with respiratory rate.

3. The patient's blood pressure and pulse should be recorded.

4. Pain should be assessed using a pain assessment tool (see page 41) to ensure effective pain relief is being achieved.

5. The level of sedation should be recorded; opiates cause sedation and it is important to ensure that the patient is still rousable.

6. The incidence/severity of nausea and vomiting should be recorded.

7. Where possible, patients' usage (i.e. how often they press the button) should be monitored to determine whether the pain control is effective.

8. The prescribed settings for the PCA system should be checked regularly to ensure proper functioning.

9. All of the above should be monitored at least hourly in the early stages. Some areas have a specially designed pain assessment tool that incorporates all of the above areas.

10. The nurse should monitor the infusion site for signs of inflammation, redness or tissue damage.

11. As with all controlled drugs, the nurse should prepare, administer and document the infusion in accordance with local trust policy.

12. The nurse should ensure no other opiates are administered whilst the patient is receiving PCA.

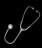

EPIDURAL ANALGESIA

Principles

Epidural analgesia is commonly used for maternal analgesia during childbirth, and patients who have undergone vascular surgery, thoracic or abdominal surgery, or orthopaedic surgery to the lower limb. It is also used for patients with intractable cancer pain and those with persistent, neuropathic or visceral pain of a chronic nature. A fine-bore catheter is inserted into the epidural space, the space between the dura mater and the ligaments and bones of the spinal cord. It can be approached at any level of the spine, but is most commonly at the lumbar or sacral level. However, the use of thoracic epidurals is increasing and is seen as the approach that demonstrates improved dynamic pain relief (Wheatley et al 2001). The catheter is usually secured to the patient's back using a sterile fixation device and a clear occlusive dressing, and is then attached to the infusion device.

The drugs most commonly used for epidural analgesia are opioids (e.g. fentanyl, diamorphine) and local anaesthetics (bupivocaine). Dosages vary according to the site of the catheter, the type of surgery, and the age and medical condition of the patient. Administration as a continuous infusion is seen as the most effective in the management of post-operative pain. Bolus injections are used less commonly for post-operative pain, but are used for the management of the pain of maternal labour. More recently, Patient Controlled Epidural Analgesia (PCEA) is being used for post-operative or persistent (chronic) pain as it affords the patient control over their analgesia. It is most effective when used in combination with a low-dose background infusion (Wheatley et al 2001).

Monitoring patients with epidural analgesia

Careful monitoring of the patient is vital and includes the following:

1. The prescribed settings on the epidural device or pump must be checked regularly to ensure it is functioning properly. The device should never be regarded as fail-safe.

2. Single luer-lock connections must be used between the catheter and the administration set. Three-way connectors must not be used to prevent inadvertent administration of other medications.

3. A bacterial filter must be in place at the end of the epidural cannula.

4. The epidural cannula must be clearly labelled.

5. The dressing over the epidural cannula site should be transparent and secure to prevent inadvertently dislodging the catheter and to minimise the risk of contamination. The inspection site should be inspected daily.

6. Close monitoring of sedation levels. Sedation and respiratory depression are known side effects of opioids. The use of a sedation score is recommended to assist in the early detection of respiratory depression. If the score signifies the patient is becoming unacceptably sedated, the infusion should be stopped and oxygen administered whilst medical or anaesthetic intervention is sought.

7. Close monitoring of respirations should be undertaken alongside sedation scores. Oxygen saturation levels are recorded with respiratory rate, although they should not be used as the primary or only indicator of respiratory depression.

8. The blood pressure and pulse rate should be recorded hourly. Hypotension is associated with the use of local anaesthetics in epidural analgesia and can also occur if the epidural catheter migrates into the subarachnoid space. This would be accompanied by light-headedness, tachycardia (raised pulse) and difficulty with movement. The infusion should be stopped and medical assistance sought immediately if any of these symptoms occur.

9. Local anaesthetics can also be toxic to the central nervous systems. The nurse should assess the patient excitation, numbness of the tongue and mouth, slurred speech, twitching, light-headedness and tinnitus (buzzing or ringing in the ears). If central nervous system toxicity occurs the patient may experience respiratory depression, convulsions and is at risk of cardiac arrest. If toxicity is suspected the infusion must be stopped. The priority of medical intervention is the patient's ventilation and oxygen needs.

10. Fluid intake should be monitored to ensure that any reduction in blood pressure is not associated with dehydration. Where possible, oral fluids must be encouraged and intravenous infusion considered.

11. Urinary output must be monitored, particularly in those patients with lumbar epidural analgesia, as it is commonly associated with urinary retention. If the patient has a urinary catheter, hourly measurements should be undertaken. Accurate recording on a fluid balance chart is essential.

12. The height of the epidural block can be assessed by the application of cold to the skin surface. If the patient reports pins and needles in the fingers this should be reported. The hourly rate of the infusion may need to be reduced.

13. Pain should be assessed using a pain assessment tool to ensure effective pain relief is being achieved. Pain should be controlled sufficiently to enable the patient to cough, breathe deeply and mobilise. If the patient reports pain at the site of the infusion, medical staff should be informed as infection or haematoma may be present.

14. Nausea and vomiting (often using a scoring system) should be recorded.

15. Patients receiving opioids can develop pruritus (itching) that is distressing and does not always respond to antihistamines. If the itching does not respond to intervention, the opioid may need to be discontinued.

16. All of the above should be monitored simultaneously and hourly for the duration of the epidural analgesia. Some areas have a specially designed assessment tool.

17. As with all controlled drugs, the nurse must prepare, administer and document the drugs according to the local policy (see page 145). No other opiates should be prescribed or administered while epidural analgesia is in progress.

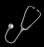

References and further reading

Temperature, pulse, respirations and blood pressure recording

Blows WT. (2001) *The biological basis of nursing: clinical observations*. Routledge, London.

This book explains the underlying physiology of all the clinical observations and what may affect the accuracy of your recordings.

Esmond G. (2001) *Respiratory nursing*. Baillière Tindall, Edinburgh.

This book provides a comprehensive resource for all aspects of respiratory nursing from the relevant A & P and respiratory assessment to smoking cessation, respiratory medication, support techniques and oxygen therapy to nutrition, pulmonary rehabilitation and end-stage management of respiratory disease.

Jevon P. (2001) Using a tympanic thermometer. *Nursing Times* **97**(9):43–44.

A useful overview of the procedure and factors that can affect the accuracy of tympanic thermometer recordings.

O'Brien E, Petrie J, Littler W. (1997) *Blood pressure measurement: recommendations of the British Hypertension Society, 3rd edn*. British Medical Journal Publishing Group, London.

Although now 10 years old it still provides an excellent guide to the correct technique for BP recording (cuff sizes, equipment, position, etc.) and the factors that can affect it. The British Hypertension Society website is also a good source of information (www.bhs.org).

Skinner S. (2005) *Understanding clinical investigations: a quick reference manual. 2nd ed.* Baillière Tindall, Edinburgh.

This excellent book provides information about a wide range of clinical investigations, including temperature, pulse respirations and BP. It includes the implications for nurses and provides a quick overview of the relevant physiology.

Care of seizures

Walker M. (2005) Status epilepticus: an evidence based guide. *BMJ* **331**:673–677.

This is an interesting article that looks at who is at risk of status epilepticus, diagnosing status epilepticus and the various drug treatments available and their benefits and side effects. Although aimed at doctors it makes interesting reading.

Cardiac monitoring and ECG

Barrett D, Gretton M, Quinn T (eds). (2006) *Cardiac care: an introduction for healthcare professionals*. John Wiley and Sons Ltd, Chichester.

This book has useful chapters on the Anatomy and physiology of the heart (Ch. 4), Assessing the cardiac patient, including ECGs (Ch. 5) and Arrhythmias (Ch. 9).

Khan E. (2004) Clinical skill: the physiological basis and interpretation of the ECG. *British Journal of Nursing* **13**(8):440–446.

This article gives a concise overview of the electrophysiology of the heart and exactly what the 12-lead ECG is looking at. It also outlines the basic rules of ECG interpretation.

Assessment of level of consciousness

Blows WT. (2001) *The biological basis of nursing: clinical observations*. Routledge, London.

Three chapters in this book explore the biological basis of neurological observations including consciousness, eyes and movement.

McLeod A. (2004) Intra- and extracranial causes of alteration in level of consciousness. *British Journal of Nursing* **13**(7):354–361.

This article examines the concepts of consciousness and intracranial pressure and what is meant by 'altered level of consciousness'. Assessment strategies are identified and AVPU, a simple alternative to the Glasgow Coma Scale, is presented as an alternative initial assessment tool.

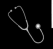
National Institute for Health and Clinical Excellence. (2003) *Head Injury: Triage, assessment, investigation and early management of head injury in infants, children and adults.* NICE, London (www.nice.org.uk).

This provides evidence-based recommendations on the management of patients with head injury. It addresses all aspects of care from pre-hospital assessment and immediate management at the scene, through assessment in A & E and admission and observation to discharge and follow-up. The document is nearly 250 pages long but it is available on the website and the recommendations are summarised from pages 6–23.

Palmer R, Knight J. (2006) Assessment of altered conscious level in clinical practice. *British Journal of Nursing* **15**(22):1255–1259.

This article critically appraises the literature focusing on the use and application of the Glasgow Coma Scale (GCS). The paper reviews the anatomical basis of consciousness and considers some of the issues of application of GCS in practice, including painful stimuli.

Price T. (2002) Painful stimuli and the Glasgow Coma Scale. *Nursing Critical Care* **7**(1):19–23.

This article presents an overview of the debate surrounding the use of painful stimuli in the use of the GCS.

Shah S. (1999) Neurological assessment (RCN Continuing Education). *Nursing Standard* **13**(22):49–56.

This article was part of the RCN Continuing Education series. It focuses on the use of the Glasgow Coma Scale and its role as part of holistic neurological assessment.

Blood glucose monitoring

Burden M. (2001) Diabetes: blood glucose monitoring. *Nursing Times* **97**(8):36–39.

This article explores why accurate technique and understanding of self-blood glucose monitoring are vital to good diabetes management.

National Institute for Clinical Excellence. (2002) *Management of type 2 diabetes – managing blood glucose levels (Guideline G).* NICE, London (www.nice.org.uk).

This guideline is part of a series of four related to the management of type 2 diabetes. Others in the series are: Retinopathy: early management and screening; Renal disease: prevention and early management; and Management of blood pressure and blood lipids.

Walker R. (2004) Capillary blood glucose monitoring and its role in diabetes management. *British Journal of Community Nursing* **9**(10):438–440.

This article explores capillary blood glucose monitoring and its role in diabetes management. Issues addressed include context and target blood glucose levels, when and by whom testing needs to be undertaken, frequency of testing, application of results, obtaining accurate and reliable results and quality control and assurance.

Pain assessment

Adams N, Field L. (2001) Pain management 1: pyschological and social aspects of pain. *British Journal of Nursing* **10**(14):903–910.

This is one of two articles in a series that examines the psychological and social factors that affect pain perception. In this article, the interactions between neurophysiological and psychological factors are outlined and theories for pain perception and ways in which the pain experience can be modulated are presented.

Broadbent C. (2000) The pharmacology of acute pain. *Nursing Times* **96**(26):39–41.

This article gives an overview of the pharmacological strategies in the management of acute pain.

Cox F. (2001) Clinical care of patients with epidural infusion. *Professional Nurse* **16**: 1429–1432.

Cox F. (2002) Making sense of epidural analgesia. *Nursing Times* **98**(32; NTPlus Pain supplement):56–58.

Both of these articles examine clinical issues related to the care of patients with epidural analgesia as well as outlining possible complications.

Davies J, McVicar A. (2000a) Issues in effective pain control 1: assessment and education. *International Journal of Palliative Nursing* **6**(2):58–65.

The first of two articles on issues related to the importance of pain assessment, the subjective nature of pain and factors such as how nurse attitudes impact on whether the patient is 'believed'. The latter part of the article addresses educational issues in the teaching and learning of pain.

Davies J, McVicar A. (2000b) Issues in effective pain control 2: from assessment to management. *International Journal of Palliative Nursing* **6**(4):162–166.

The second article addresses the problem of nurses' attitudes and belief with regard to self-assessment of pain and suggests that the most effective way to prevent barriers arising is to ensure nurses receive input on pain assessment and pain control in their preregistration studies.

Duke S. (2006) Pain. In: Alexander MF, Fawcett JN, Runciman PJ (eds). *Nursing Practice Hospital and Home*. Churchill Livingstone, Edinburgh.

This chapter presents an overview of all aspects of pain including the experience of pain, mechanisms of pain, theories of pain, key concepts, pain management and barriers to pain management.

Field L, Adams N. (2001) Pain management 2: the use of psychological approaches to pain. *British Journal of Nursing* **10**(15):971–974.

The second of two articles that examine the importance of the nurse–patient interaction in the management of patients' pain. It outlines the adoption of several psychological approaches that could be used by nurses when dealing with patients in pain.

Lynch M. (2001) Pain as the fifth vital sign. *Journal of Intravenous Nursing* **24**(2):85–94.

This article explores the importance of assessing and monitoring patients' pain.

Macintyre PE. (2001) Safety and efficacy of patient-controlled analgesia. *British Journal of Anaesthesia* **87**(1):36–46.

This article explores a range of safety and efficacy issues associated with patient-controlled analgesia including analgesic efficacy, analgesic use, patient outcomes, patient factors, equipment factors, medical and nursing staff factors and the PCA prescription.

McCaffery M, Ferrell BR. (1997) Nurses' knowledge of pain assessment and management: how much progress have we made? *Journal of Pain and Symptom Management* **14**(3):175–188.

This article argues that improvements in nurses' knowledge of pain assessment, opioid dosing and the likelihood of addiction seem to be evident from a review of surveys in 1995 and compared with similar surveys conducted in 1988. However, knowledge deficits related to the importance of patients' self-reports of pain and fear of addiction in certain circumstances remain. Although now 10 years old, the issues raised remain as relevant today.

Pasero C. (2003) Epidural analgesia for postoperative pain. *American Journal of Nursing* **103**(10):62–64.

This article presents an overview of the benefits of epidural analgesia for the management of post-operative pain. Epidural anatomy, methods of administration, characteristics of epidural opioids, combining local anaesthetics and opioids and traditional pain management versus epidural analgesia are all addressed in a brief way.

Pasero C, McCaffery M. (2006) Safe use of continuous infusion with IV PCA. *Journal of PeriAnaesthesia Nursing* **19**(1):42–45.

This article primarily addresses the issues of safety in the use of a background continuous infusion with an intravenous PCA. The article concludes that the practice is controversial and caution must be exercised particularly with opioid-naïve patients. With appropriate safety measures the practice is deemed to be effective.

Wheatley R, Schug S, Watson D. (2001) Safety and efficacy of postoperative epidural analgesia. *British Journal of Anaesthesia* **87**(1):47–61.

This article examines issues of safety and efficacy in the use of post-operative epidural analgesia. Efficacy issues include the choice of drug, site of insertion, pre- or post-incisional epidural analgesia and method of drug delivery. Safety issues addressed include incidence of neurological complications due to epidural analgesia, adverse events due to insertion of needle and catheter, adverse events due to the presence of an indwelling catheter in the epidural space, adverse events related to epidural drug administration and organisational issues.

White S. (2004) Assessment of chronic neuropathic pain and the use of pain tools. *British Journal of Nursing* **13**(7):372–378.

This article examines the evidence base for the assessment of chronic neuropathic pain and discusses some of the main tools and their suitability for use for this particular type of pain.

2

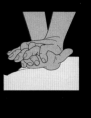

Resuscitation

ASSESSMENT OF A COLLAPSED PERSON (OUT OF HOSPITAL)

Preparation

Patient	Equipment/Environment	Nurse
• The person is unresponsive when called or shaken.	• No equipment is necessary.	• Behave calmly.

Procedure PFP1

Danger

1. Approach the person/surroundings carefully to exclude any risk of danger to yourself, e.g. electrical cable. There may be something to indicate the possible cause of collapse (e.g. fall or injury). Kneel beside the person.

Response

2. Assess the person's conscious state. Shake their shoulders (unless possible neck injury) and shout (in both ears) to see if they respond.

Assistance

3. If the person is unconscious (i.e. totally unresponsive) call for help from a bystander (if present). Ask the bystander to wait while you complete your assessment. If you are completely alone *do not* go for help yourself at this stage.

Airway

4. With one hand tip back the forehead (unless neck injury) and with two fingers of your other hand lift the chin to raise the tongue from the back of the throat to open the airway (see Figure 2.3). Look for any obstruction in the mouth. Keep the chin raised.

Breathing

5. Place your cheek near the person's nostrils to **feel** for any breathing. **Look** for chest movement and **listen** for breath sounds. Observe for no more than 10 seconds. If breathing is present, place the casualty in the recovery position (Figure 2.1). If no breathing is detected, start basic life support (see page 54).

Recovery position

1. Continue to kneel beside the person.

2. If the person is wearing spectacles remove these and place on one side PFP2.

3. Position the person's nearest arm at 90° to their shoulder with the elbow bent.

4. Hold the back of the person's other hand against their cheek that is nearest to you and keep holding it in position.

5. Take hold of the leg furthest from you at the knee and raise it until the foot is flat on the floor.

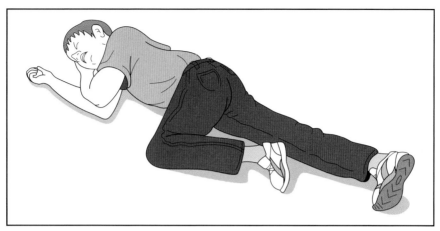

Figure 2.1 Recovery position

6. Place your hand on the knee and pull towards you so that the person turns onto their side **PFP3**.

7. Draw the person's knee towards their chest to prevent them rolling onto their stomach.

8. Tilt the chin again to maintain an open airway.

9. Send for help **PFP4** and continue to observe the person closely to ensure that breathing and circulation are being maintained.

10. If the ambulance has not arrived by 30 minutes, turn the person to their other side to prevent pressure ulcers.

Points for practice

1. The mnemonic DR ABC (Doctor ABC – Danger, Response, Assistance, Airway, Breathing and Circulation) will help you remember the procedure for assessing a collapsed person. Resuscitation guidelines are reviewed regularly; it is important to check the Resuscitation Council website regularly for the most recent guidance.

2. Spectacles may get broken and cause discomfort when the person is turned onto their side in the recovery position.

3. Before turning the person onto their side check to see that there is nothing large in the pocket (e.g. large bunch of keys) that might cause damage if lying on it for a period of time.

4. If the collapse has occurred in the street or someone's home, send for an ambulance. If it is in a hospital or nursing home, refer to local policy. At this point you can go for help yourself if no one else is available.

BASIC LIFE SUPPORT

Preparation

Patient	Equipment/Environment	Nurse
• The patient is unresponsive when called or shaken.	• Some people carry a pocket resuscitation mask, which may be used to prevent contact with the person's saliva during mouth-to-mouth respiration in an emergency (**Figure 2.2**). Some nursing homes/clinics also make these available.	• Yearly updating in resuscitation techniques is vital to maintain these skills. • Resuscitation guidelines are reviewed regularly; it is important to check the Resuscitation Council website regularly for the most recent guidance.

Procedure

Danger

1. Approach the person/surroundings carefully to exclude any risk of danger to yourself, e.g. electrical cable. There may be something to indicate the possible cause of collapse (e.g. fall or injury). Kneel beside the person.

Response

2. Assess the person's conscious state. Shake their shoulders (unless possible neck injury) and shout (in both ears) to see if they respond.

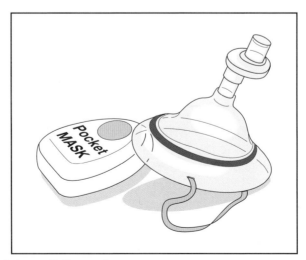

Figure 2.2 Pocket resuscitation mask

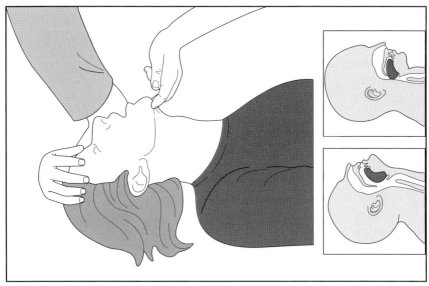

Figure 2.3 Chin lifted to bring tongue forward from back of throat

Assistance

3. If the person is unconscious (i.e. totally unresponsive) call for help from a bystander (if present). Ask the bystander to wait while you complete your assessment. If you are completely alone *do not* go for help yourself at this stage.

Airway

4. With one hand tip back the forehead (unless neck injury) and with two fingers of your other hand lift the chin to raise the tongue from the back of the throat to open the airway (see Figure 2.3). Look for any obstruction in the mouth. Keep the chin raised.

Breathing

5. Place your cheek near the person's nostrils to **feel** for any breathing. **Look** for chest movement and **listen** for breath sounds. Observe for no more than 10 seconds.

6. If the person is **not breathing** normally send for help (or go yourself if no one else is around) PFP1 and then commence cardiopulmonary resuscitation (CPR, see below) PFP2.

CARDIOPULMONARY RESUSCITATION

1. With the person lying flat on their back commence external cardiac compressions.

2. **Hand position.** Identify the middle of the sternum (breast bone) and place the heel of one hand in the middle of the lower half of the sternum. Place your other hand on top and interlock the fingers (see Figure 2.4) **PFP3**.

3. Keeping your arms straight and your shoulders in line with your elbows and heels of your hands give 30 compressions at a rate of approximately 100 per minute. You should press hard enough to compress the chest wall by 4–5 cm (Resuscitation Council UK 2005 – **PFP4**).

4. **Mouth-to-mouth breathing.** Keeping the chin lifted, pinch the soft part of the person's nose. Take a normal breath in and place your lips around the person's open mouth and ensure a good seal. Blow steadily into the person's mouth whilst watching from the corner of your eye to see the chest rise. Take your mouth away as the chest falls and air comes out. Repeat once **PFP5**.

5. Continue giving cycles of 30 compressions and two breaths until help arrives **PFP6**.

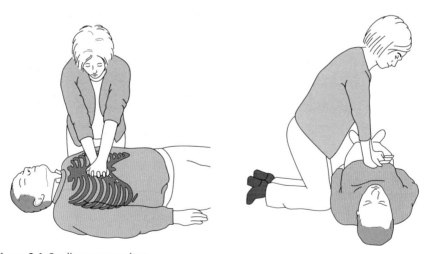

Figure 2.4 Cardiac compressions

Post procedure

Patient

- Once help arrives, the experienced professionals will take over from you.

Nurse

- Cardiopulmonary resuscitation is physically and emotionally exhausting. Try to talk through what happened with someone afterwards.
- Despite your best efforts, the person may not survive.

Points for practice

1. If there is no-one to send for help it is important to go yourself before you start cardiopulmonary resuscitation so that help will be on its way. However, it is important to check the airway and breathing before you do so (see step 3).

2. Feel for the carotid pulse if you have been trained to do so and look for general signs of circulation such as movement, coughing, groaning, etc. The carotid pulse is nearest to the heart. If no pulse can be felt here, there is no cardiac output. If this is a respiratory arrest (i.e. circulation is present, but the person is not breathing) go to step 4 and give 10 breaths per minute.

3. The person's outer clothing may need to be removed to ensure the correct positioning of the hands.

4. Resuscitation procedures are reviewed regularly. It is important to ensure that you have knowledge of the most up-to-date guidelines.

5. The chest should rise with every breath. If it does not, check the mouth again for visible obstruction and make sure the chin is still lifted to bring the tongue forward. Do not over-breathe as this may inflate the stomach and cause vomiting. Wait for the chest to fall after each breath before giving another breath.

6. If more than one person is present alternate between compressions and mouth-to-mouth breathing every 2 minutes.

WARD-BASED CARDIOPULMONARY RESUSCITATION

Preparation

Patient

Check:

- Unconscious
- Not breathing
- No pulse
- Is the patient for resuscitation? `PFP1`.

Equipment/Environment

- Emergency equipment box or trolley including emergency drugs box `PFP2`.
- Gloves, goggles and plastic aprons (usually kept with emergency equipment).
- Oxygen cylinder (if piped oxygen is not available).
- Suction machine (if piped suction is not available).
- Intravenous infusion stand.
- Cardiac monitor and defibrillator.
- Screen bed area to maintain privacy `PFP3`.

Nurse

- Summon help `PFP4`.
- The most experienced nurse should co-ordinate the activities of other staff.
- If sufficient staff is available, delegate someone to care for the other patients.

Procedure

1. Lay the patient flat. If in bed, remove pillows and the head of the bed `PFP5`.
2. If there is no carotid pulse, commence cardiopulmonary resuscitation at a ratio of 30 compressions to two breaths (see page 56).
3. Once available, insert an appropriate sized oropharyngeal (Guedel) airway `PFP6`. Insert it into the mouth upside down and then turn it into position over the back of the tongue (Figure 2.5).
4. Attach the oxygen tubing to the mask/valve bag (e.g. Ambu bag) and set oxygen flow to 10 l per minute `PFP7`.
5. Holding the chin up and the face mask tight against the face (Figure 2.6), compress the bag at a steady speed. Check that the chest is rising with each compression of the bag `PFP8`.
6. Continue giving 30 external cardiac compressions to every 2 'breaths'.
7. When the medical/senior nursing team arrives the following may be instigated according to the condition of the patient:
   - Endotracheal intubation – check the suction machine is working and has an oral (Yankauer) sucker attached. Once the patient is intubated, a tracheal suction catheter will be required.
   - Intravenous cannulation (often internal/external jugular) to enable drugs such as epinephrine (adrenaline) to be given intravenously.
   - Cardiac monitoring/recording.
   - Defibrillation.
8. The timing of each event and the administration of any drugs must be documented.

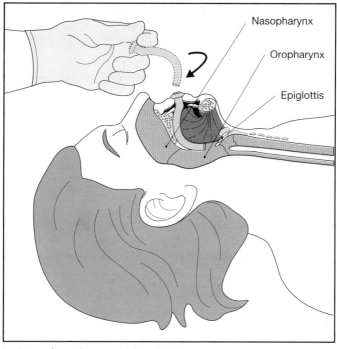

Nasopharynx

Oropharynx

Epiglottis

Figure 2.5 Position of oropharyngeal (Guedel) airway

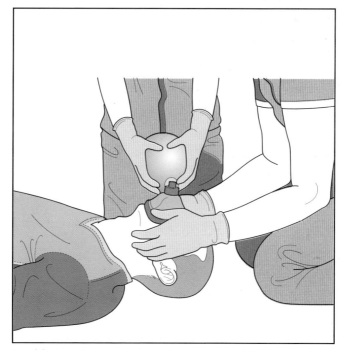

Figure 2.6 Use of face mask and valve/mask bag

Post procedure

Patient	Equipment/Environment	Nurse
• If resuscitation is successful, close monitoring of the patient's condition will be necessary. The patient may be transferred to an intensive care unit.	• Emergency equipment must be cleaned and restocked immediately and made ready for use.	• Document the event in the patient's records.
• If resuscitation is unsuccessful, ensure privacy and dignity are maintained and prepare the patient to be seen by the family **PFP9**.	• Dispose of used equipment according to local policy.	• All involved should discuss the way the situation was managed **PFP10**.

Points for practice

1. Resuscitation is not appropriate in some patients. The situation must be discussed with the patient and/or the family and if a decision has been made not to resuscitate, this must be written in the medical notes by the patient's medical consultant. It should also be written in the nursing documentation and communicated at every shift handover.

2. When starting work or placement in a new clinical area it is important to note the location of emergency equipment and the emergency telephone numbers.

3. If this is not easily achieved then screen other patients to ensure privacy and reduce their distress at seeing what is happening.

4. In a hospital, there will be a Resuscitation Team, who can be summoned urgently by phoning a special number. It is vital to check that you know the emergency number in every area that you work. The ward may also have an emergency buzzer system to summon help.

5. If this is a witnessed cardiac arrest a skilled professional may deliver a precordial thump (Jevon 2006). If the patient is on a pressure-relieving mattress, it will have a quick-release mechanism to enable rapid deflation in an emergency.

6. The Guedel airway is designed to hold the tongue forward to prevent it obstructing the airway. The correct size is determined by choosing an airway that is the same length as the distance from the tip of the patient's ear to the corner of his/her mouth.

7. Oxygen may be given without prescription in an emergency situation.

8. Two people will be required for this; one to hold the face mask in position and the other to squeeze the Ambu bag.

9. Make sure that all the equipment has been cleared away and that the bed area is tidy. One pillow should be placed under the head and the bed made as usual with sheets and a counterpane.

10. If the resuscitation is unsuccessful, it can be distressing for all involved and time should be made available to support junior staff and talk it through.

References and further reading

Gallimore D. (2006) Understanding the drugs used during cardiac arrest response. *Nursing Times* **102**(23):24–26.

  A useful guide to the drugs used in a cardiac arrest and how they work.

Jevon P. (2006) Resuscitation skills part 1: Recovery position. *Nursing Times* **102**(25):28–29.

Jevon P. (2006) Resuscitation skills part 2: Clearing the airway. *Nursing Times* **102**(26): 26–27.

Jevon P. (2006) Resuscitation skills part 3: Basic airway management. *Nursing Times* **102**(28):26–27.

Jevon P. (2006) Resuscitation skills part 4: Chest compressions. *Nursing Times* **102**(28): 26–27.

  This clearly written series of articles gives an overview of the whole resuscitation procedure with detailed discussion and clear diagrams to show each stage.

Jevon P. (2006) Resuscitation skills part 5: Precordial thump. *Nursing Times* **102**(29):28–29.

  This article discusses the use of the precordial thump, which should be considered when cardiac arrest is witnessed and a defibrillator is not readily available, but only by professionals who have been specifically trained in its use (Resuscitation Council UK 2005).

Moule P, Albarran J. (2005) *Practical resuscitation, recognition and response*. Blackwell Publishing, Oxford.

  An excellent resource that covers all aspects of resuscitation including professional and ethical/legal issues, recognising the sick patient and preventing cardiac arrest, BLS and advanced resuscitation, and post-resuscitation care.

Website

Resuscitation Council UK. Resuscitation Guidelines 2005. Resuscitation Council London. www.resus.org.uk

  This website has the most up-to-date guidelines and you should check it regularly for updates.

Notes

3

Intravenous therapy

VENEPUNCTURE

Preparation

Patient	Equipment/Environment	Nurse
• Explain the procedure, to gain consent and co-operation.	• Green needle (21G) and syringe (size will vary according to the amount of blood needed) and blood sample tubes as appropriate, or vacuum tube sampling system and appropriate sample tubes.	• Hands must be washed and dried thoroughly.
• The patient should be sitting or lying comfortably, with the appropriate arm supported.		• Gloves (close-fitting to allow dexterity) should be worn.
• If clothing is tight or restrictive remove the arm from the sleeve.	• Skin-cleansing agent.	• Additional protective clothing may be necessary if indicated by the patient's condition (see Chapter 9).
	• Tourniquet.	
	• Gauze swabs or cotton-wool balls.	
	• Small self-adhesive dressing.	
	• Sharps bin.	

Procedure

1. Check the patient's identity with the blood test request form and ask/assist patient to adjust clothing as necessary.

2. Assemble all equipment. Do not label the sample tubes until the blood specimen is in them PFP1.

3. Inspect the arm to select a suitable vein PFP2 and apply the tourniquet PFP3. Palpate the vein to locate its position and ensure that it is not an artery (which will pulsate) or a tendon.

4. Clean the skin with the skin-cleansing agent and allow it to dry completely PFP4.

5. With the patient's arm straight and well supported, use your non-dominant hand to pull the skin tight over the vein to 'anchor' the vein.

6. Take the syringe and needle (or needle and plastic holder of vacuum system) in your dominant hand. With the bevel of the needle upward and directly over the vein, insert the needle at an angle of about 15° through the skin and into the vein.

7. **Needle and syringe** – blood will appear at the tip of the syringe to indicate that the vein has been punctured. Hold the needle in position with one hand and, with the other, steadily pull back the piston of the syringe until the required amount of blood is obtained (Figure 3.1A). Do not pull too vigorously or the vein may collapse.
   Vacuum system – after puncturing the vein, no blood is visible until the sample tube is attached. Hold the needle and plastic holder securely in place

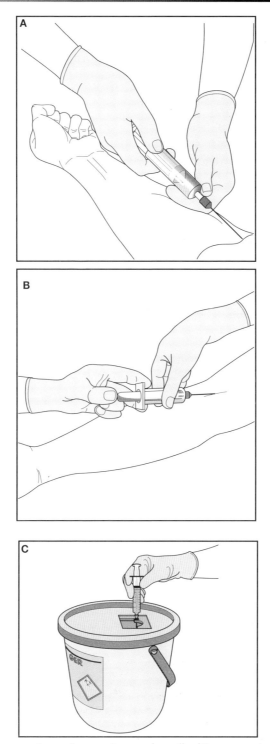

Figure 3.1 (A) Venepuncture using a syringe and needle, (B) venepuncture using a vacuum system, (C) using the non-touch needle removing device

and attach the sample tube by pushing it firmly onto the needle attachment inside the holder (**Figure 3.1B**). The tube will then automatically fill with blood to the required amount. If additional samples are required, remove the tube when full (no blood will leak out) and attach another.

8. Remove the tourniquet, hold the gauze swab or cotton-wool ball over the puncture site and remove the needle. Do not press until the needle is out of the vein as this is very painful for the patient. Continue to apply pressure (or ask the patient to do this) for 2–3 minutes until the bleeding stops, to prevent bruising.

9. **Needle and syringe** – using the non-touch needle-removing device on the sharps bin (**Figure 3.1C**), remove the needle from the syringe before transferring the blood to the sample tube PFP5.
   Vacuum system – using the non-touch needle-removing device on the sharps bin (**Figure 3.1C**). Remove the needle and discard. If appropriate, retain the plastic holder for future use PFP6.

Post procedure

Patient	Equipment/Environment	Nurse
• Ask the patient to continue pressing but not to bend the arm as this may cause a haematoma. Once the bleeding has stopped, apply a small self-adhesive dressing. • Assist the patient to replace clothing as necessary.	• Discard all sharps and other waste safely.	• Remove gloves and wash hands. • Label specimens with the patient's surname, first names, hospital number, date of birth, ward/clinic and the date of the sample.

Points for practice

1. Do not label the sample tubes in advance in case venepuncture is unsuccessful and the tubes are mistakenly used for another patient.

2. The best veins are usually found at the elbow, in the antecubital fossa. These veins are less mobile, easier to puncture and less painful than veins in the hand or lower arm. If the patient is very cold, it may help to ask the patient to warm their hands in warm water for a few minutes or clench and unclench a fist several times to increase blood flow to the arm. Gently tapping the vein may also increase vasodilation by causing histamine release at the site. This must be gentle as vigorous tapping may cause venous spasm.

3. The tourniquet should not be applied for longer than 1 minute before collecting the blood specimen. Prolonged use will cause intravascular fluid to leak into the tissues and may affect the accuracy of the blood test (Lavery & Ingram 2005).

4. The skin-cleansing agent is usually alcohol-based and must be allowed to dry completely before proceeding. Any residual alcohol causes pain for the patient and may damage the cells and affect the blood specimen.

5. Cells may be damaged if the blood is squirted through the needle into the sample tube. Damage can cause them to leak potassium and may lead to an inaccurate result.

6. Refer to local policy regarding re-use of the plastic holder. It should always be discussed if it becomes contaminated with blood or the patient has an infection such as hepatitis or MRSA.

INTRAVENOUS CANNULATION

Preparation

Patient

- Explain the procedure, to gain consent and co-operation.
- The patient should be sitting or lying comfortably, with the appropriate arm (non-dominant if possible) supported. If the cannula is for an intravenous infusion or the clothing is tight or restrictive, remove the arm from the sleeve.
- Local anaesthetic cream, if used, must be applied at least 1 hour prior to the procedure PFP1.
- Cannulation will be easier if the patient's arms and hands are warm and well perfused.

Equipment/Environment

- Tourniquet.
- Skin-cleansing agent (e.g. chlorhexidine in alcohol) according to local policy.
- Cannula of appropriate size PFP2 – check the expiry date and that the packaging is intact.
- Sterile cannula dressing according to local policy PFP3.
- Ten millilitres of 0.9% sodium chloride to flush the cannula (check the expiry date).
- Injectable cap or prepared infusion ready to connect (see page 72).
- Disposable pad or towel to place under the arm to protect the bed linen.
- Sharps bin.
- Environment should ensure warmth, privacy and adequate lighting.

Nurse

- Hands must be washed and dried thoroughly.
- Gloves (close-fitting to allow dexterity) and an apron should be worn.
- Additional protective clothing may be necessary if indicated by the patient's condition (see Chapter 9).

Procedure

1. If possible, choose the patient's non-dominant arm for cannulation. Place towel or pad under the arm.

2. Apply the tourniquet 5–10 cm above the proposed site of cannulation PFP4 and check for arterial blood flow. If the tourniquet is so tight that it prevents arterial blood flow, the veins will not fill.

3. Ask the patient to clench and unclench their fist several times to encourage venous filling. Gently tapping the vein may also encourage vasodilation by causing histamine release at the site. Select a vein by palpation, not just visually, to ensure that it is suitable (i.e. bouncy not hard) and is not an artery (which will pulsate) or a tendon PFP5.

4. Clean the site with cleansing agent and allow it to dry. Do not touch the site again with your fingers.

5. Take the cannula and check that the needle can be removed easily, but do not remove it. Hold the cannula in your dominant hand with the sharp bevelled end facing upwards (Figure 3.2).

6. With your other hand, hold the patient's arm and 'anchor' the vein with your thumb, just below the selected insertion site, to prevent it moving when punctured.

7. Holding the cannula at an angle of 20–30° either directly over the vein or just to one side of it, insert the cannula through the skin and into the vein **PFP6**.

8. Stop advancing the cannula as soon as blood appears at the end of the cannula, which indicates that it has entered the vein and lower the angle of the cannula.

9. Holding the needle part of the cannula with one hand to stop it advancing any further (and going right through the vein), slide the cannula off the needle and into the vein with the other hand.

10. Hold the cannula in place to prevent dislodgement and release the tourniquet. Place a piece of sterile gauze under the end of the cannula to contain any drops of blood during removal of the needle (step 13).

11. If an injectable cap is being used, open the packaging (taking care not to contaminate the sterile end) and hold it between the thumb and forefinger of your dominant hand. If an infusion is to be connected omit this step and follow the procedure in 'Preparing an infusion', see page 72.

12. With your other hand, apply pressure to the vein immediately above the end of the cannula to minimise blood flow (Figure 3.3).

13. Remove the needle and swiftly insert the injectable cap or the administration set of the infusion.

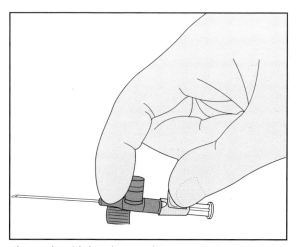

Figure 3.2 Winged cannula with bevel upwards

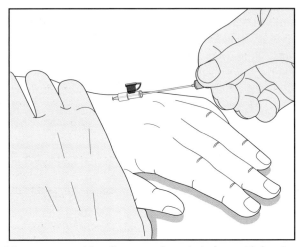

Figure 3.3 Applying pressure with a finger on the vein before withdrawing the needle

14. Clean up any blood and apply the sterile dressing **PFP7**, ensuring that the cannula is held securely in place.
15. Flush the cannula with 0.9% sodium chloride to ensure patency.

Post procedure

Patient
- Explain any restrictions to mobility and the need to protect the cannula site.
- Instruct the patient to report any swelling, redness or pain.

Equipment/Environment
- Discard sharps and other clinical waste safely.
- Return sharps bin and tourniquet to the appropriate places.

Nurse
- Remove gloves and apron and wash hands.
- Document the date and time of cannulation in the nursing records.

Points for practice

1. Although most adult patients will not require it, local anaesthetic may be desirable with patients who are extremely anxious or needle-phobic. Local anaesthetic cream must be applied at least 1 hour in advance to be effective and the possibility of allergy must be considered. The use of injected local anaesthetic is debatable as this requires a needle-prick and may make the selected vein more difficult to see (Lavery & Ingram 2005).

2. The size of cannula required will be determined by the type of fluid to be infused and the size and condition of the patient's veins. The smallest gauge capable of achieving the required flow rate should be used (RCN 2003).

3. The dressing must be sterile. Transparent semi-permeable membrane dressings and those that are gauze and transparent membrane are ideal as they permit visual inspection of the site without removal of the dressing.

4. Site selection should avoid areas of flexion if at all possible and the distal areas of the upper limbs should routinely be used first. This allows subsequent cannulation to proximal to the previously cannulated site (RCN 2003).

5. If it is difficult to palpate the vein with gloves on, do this without gloves and then put them on once the vein is identified.

6. Despite 'anchoring' with the thumb, the vein sometimes moves when directly punctured from above. Consequently, many people prefer to insert the cannula through the skin slightly to one side of the vein and then direct it into the vein.

7. The type of dressing used will be dictated by local policy. Non-sterile tape should not be used to secure the cannula as this has been shown to increase the risk of infection.

PREPARING AN INFUSION

Preparation

Patient

- Explain the reasons for intravenous infusion and any limitations to mobility.

Equipment/Environment

- Intravenous infusion fluid according to the prescription.
- Intravenous administration set of appropriate type **PFP1**.
- Intravenous infusion stand.
- Sterile gauze squares.

Nurse

- Wash and dry hands thoroughly.
- Gloves should be worn when connecting the infusion to the cannula.
- Additional protective clothing may be necessary if indicated by the patient's condition (see Chapter 9).

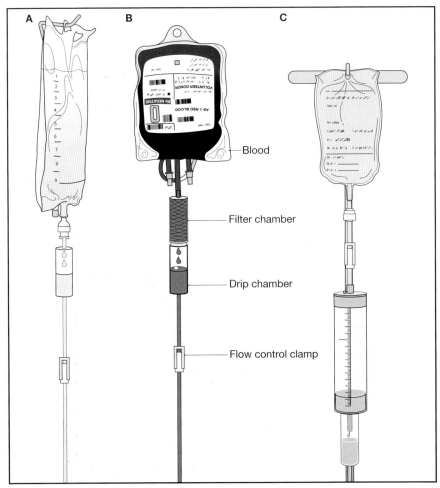

Figure 3.4 (A) Standard administration set, (B) blood administration set, (C) burette

Procedure

Intravenous fluid

1. The intravenous fluid to be administered must be checked by a registered nurse **PFP2**. Blood transfusions require special checking procedure (see page 100).
2. Check the outer wrapper is intact and not damaged in any way.
3. Open the outer wrapper and remove the bag.
4. Check the fluid bag for leakage, particles, cloudiness, expiry date and batch number.

Administration set

1. Check the contents are sterile, i.e. the outer wrapper is not damaged or wet.
2. Check the expiry date/date of sterilisation.
3. Open the packaging and remove the administration set. Both ends should be covered with protective caps to maintain sterility.
4. Close the flow control clamp on the administration set.

Assembly

1. Remove the protective cap from the insertion port on the bag of fluid and hold carefully to maintain sterility.
2. Remove the protective cover from the spike of the administration set (just above the drip chamber).
3. Taking care to maintain sterility, insert the spike into the bag, pushing and twisting until fully inserted (see Figure 3.5).
4. Hang the bag on the infusion stand. Squeeze and release the drip chamber until it is half-full of fluid.

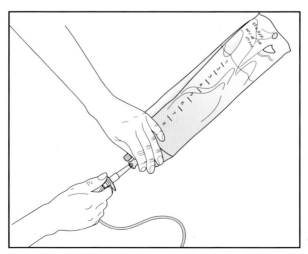

Figure 3.5 Inserting the spike of the administration set into the infusion bag

5. To expel the air from the administration set, partially open the roller clamp to allow fluid to run through the set; not too quickly or it will draw in air from the drip chamber.

6. When all the air has been expelled, close the roller clamp. The infusion is now ready for use (Figure 3.6).

Connecting the infusion

7. Put on gloves and place a folded gauze square under the end of the cannula to catch any spillage.

8. Taking care to maintain sterility, remove the protective cap from the administration set and the cap from the cannula. Swiftly connect the set and 'lock' into position **PFP4**.

9. Secure the tubing with tape to prevent pulling (see Figure 3.7 on page 75) and adjust the roller clamp to set the infusion to the prescribed rate (see page 76).

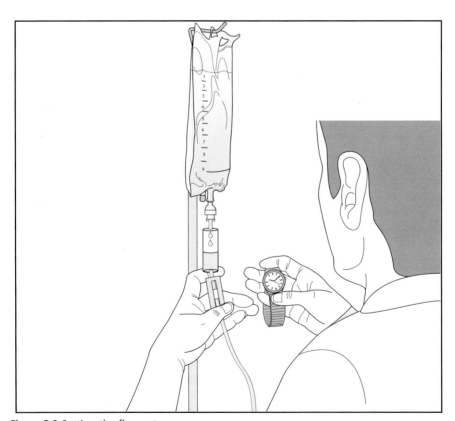

Figure 3.6 Setting the flow rate

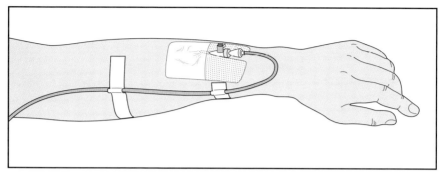

Figure 3.7 Securing the intravenous tubing

Post procedure

Patient	Equipment/Environment	Nurse
• Ensure the patient is comfortable and understands about the infusion.	• Discard all packaging into the clinical waste system.	• Remove gloves and wash hands.
• Instruct the patient to report any swelling, redness or pain.		• Record the time the infusion started and the batch number of the intravenous fluid according to local policy.
		• Document the care in the nursing records.

Points for practice

1. The type of administration set used will depend upon the type of fluid being administered. Blood requires an administration set with a filter (Figure 3.4B) that incorporates a 170 mm filter to remove microaggregates that are formed during storage of the blood (Bradbury & Cruickshank 2000). Clear fluids require a simple administration set without a filter chamber (Figure 3.4A).

2. In most cases, all intravenous fluids must be checked by a registered nurse, although this may vary according to local policy. In some Trusts, two nurses are required to check intravenous fluid. Procedures for checking blood transfusions are detailed on page 100.

3. Infusions requiring great accuracy will be controlled through an intravenous pump or syringe driver. A burette (Figure 3.4C) may be used to administer small amounts of fluid or drugs.

4. All administration sets should be fitted with a luer lock device that can be twisted to lock the tubing in place. This is to prevent an accidental disconnection and prevent the entry of micro-organisms. Replacing administration sets every 72 hours has been shown to be safe; however, they should be changed more frequently if used to administer blood (see page 104) or parenteral nutrition (see page 96).

CHANGING AN INFUSION BAG

Preparation

Patient	Equipment/Environment	Nurse
• Explain the procedure.	• Intravenous infusion fluid as prescribed.	• The hands must be washed and dried thoroughly.
	• For blood transfusions see page 100.	• The infusion fluid must be checked by a registered nurse.

Procedure

1. Remove the infusion fluid from its outer wrapper and check the fluid bag for leakage, particles, cloudiness, expiry date, volume and batch number.

2. Ensure that it is the correct infusion fluid by checking it with the prescription chart and the patient's identity. (NB This must be checked by a registered nurse, see page 75.)

3. Close the roller clamp on the administration set.

4. Remove the empty infusion bag from the stand and pull out the spike of the administration set, taking care not to contaminate it.

5. Remove the protective cover from the inlet port of the new infusion bag and insert the spike of the giving set, twisting until fully inserted (Figure 3.5).

6. Replace the bag on the infusion stand and adjust the roller clamp to the prescribed flow rate (see page 78).

Post procedure

Patient	Equipment/Environment	Nurse
• Check at least hourly that the infusion is running as prescribed and the patient is not complaining of pain or discomfort at the site.	• Discard the used infusion bag and packaging into the clinical waste system **PFP1**.	• Document the infusion (amount, type of fluid, time commenced, batch number and signature of the nurse) according to local policy.
• Observe the patient for signs of fluid overload (rising pulse and respiratory rate).		• If the patient has a fluid chart, the infusion should be recorded on this according to local policy **PFP2**.

Points for practice

1. If changing the administration set as well as the bag, the spike of the set should be discarded into a sharps bin.

2. Most patients with an intravenous infusion will require a fluid balance chart to monitor fluid input and output (see page 190). The new infusion and completion of the old infusion should be recorded.

REGULATION OF FLOW RATE

Principles

The use of intravenous devices (pumps and syringe drivers) to regulate infusions is steadily increasing. However, a large number of simple infusions will be regulated using gravity and the roller clamp only (Figure 3.6). It is important that infusions run at a constant rate over the prescribed time.

Calculating the flow rate in 'drops per minute'

If it is a simple gravity infusion, or an infusion device that regulates the flow rate in 'drops per minute' is being used, calculation of the rate in drops per minute is necessary **PFP1**. The calculation is as follows:

$$\frac{\text{volume of infusion in ml} \times \text{number of drops per ml}}{\text{time in minutes}}$$

$$= \text{flow rate in drops per minute}$$

The number of drops per ml will be determined by the administration set being used and is indicated on the packaging **PFP2**:

- Standard administration set = 20 drops per ml.
- Blood administration set = 15 drops per ml.
- Paediatric set (burette) = 60 drops per ml.

Example: A patient has been prescribed 500 ml of 0.9% sodium chloride (normal saline) to be given over 6 hours using a standard administration set. The calculation is as follows:

$$\frac{\textbf{500}(\text{vol. of infusion}) \times 20(\text{No. of drops per ml})}{\textbf{360}(6 \text{ hours} \times 60 \text{ minutes})} = \frac{500 \times 20}{360} = \frac{10\,000}{360}$$

$$= \textbf{27.77 drops per minute} \text{ (round up to 28 drops)}$$

Example: A patient has been prescribed 420 ml of whole blood to be given over 4 hours using a blood administration set. The calculation is as follows:

$$\frac{420 \times 15}{240} = \frac{6300}{240} = \textbf{26.25 drops per minute} \text{ (round up to 27 drops)}$$

Calculating the flow rate in 'millilitres per hour'

$$\frac{\text{volume of infusion in ml}}{\text{No. of hours}} = \text{flow rate in millilitres per hour}$$

Example: A patient has been prescribed 1 litre of 5% dextrose to be given over 8 hours. The calculation is as follows:

$$\frac{1000}{8} = \textbf{125 ml per hour}$$

Points for practice

1. You are likely to be using a calculator for these calculations. It is important to check your answer several times to ensure that you have used the correct maths. If you are working with junior nurses, it is important to be able to demonstrate your calculation, to enable them to learn.

2. A packaging of a blood administration set may state that it gives 20 drops per ml, but this relates to drops of water. Because blood is thicker than water it forms a larger drop and there are only 15 drops to each ml.

INTRAVENOUS PUMPS AND SYRINGE DRIVERS

Principles

Intravenous pumps and syringe drivers are increasingly being used to control infusions in general wards as well as in specialist areas. There are a large number of different types available from a range of manufacturers and a detailed description of each will be found in the manufacturer's users' manual. To guarantee safe and accurate practice, nurses have a responsibility to ensure that they are familiar with any equipment being used. If unsure of any aspect of the pump or syringe driver, it is important to seek help from a more experienced nurse or from the hospital department where intravenous devices are maintained. Although intravenous devices may differ in appearance, there are a number of features that are likely to be common to all. Make sure you are familiar with the following features on the syringe driver or pump you are using.

Power supply

- Is the device powered by battery, mains electricity or both?
- If batteries, what type are they?
- If it has a rechargeable battery: how long will it run on the battery?; how is the battery charged?; how do you know when it needs charging?

Administration set/cassette/syringe

- Most devices can only be used with a specific administration set, cassette or type of syringe.
- If it is possible to use different sizes and types, how does the device confirm recognition of the type being used?

Setting up the device

- You must be familiar with the correct procedure for setting up the device. All administration sets, cassettes and syringes are designed to be inserted easily into the device. If force is required, the correct procedure is not being followed.

Alarm systems

- Most devices have a number of alarms to alert the nurse to situations such as 'air in the line', 'infusion complete' and 'occlusion of the line'.
- Most will have a mute button to allow the alarm to be silenced while dealing with the problem. It is vital that alarms are never turned off (however irritating), as dangerous situations may then go undetected.
- If any alarm feature is not working properly, the device must not be used.
- Some smaller devices do not have any alarms and must be checked at least once every hour to ensure safe and accurate administration of the drug or infusion.

Maintenance and repair

- All intravenous devices must be maintained regularly to ensure safe and accurate use. Most hospitals have a system of regular maintenance indicated by a sticker on the device, showing the date when maintenance is due. Pumps and syringe drivers must not be used after this date and should be returned to the relevant department for maintenance.

• Most devices that are powered by mains electricity also have a battery for short-term use when transferring a patient or during a power cut. The device should be kept plugged in to the mains at all times, even when not in use, to ensure the battery remains fully charged.

CARE OF PERIPHERAL CANNULA SITE

Preparation

Patient

- Inspect the cannula site to determine whether the dressing needs changing `PFP1`.
- Explain the procedure, to gain consent and co-operation.
- The patient must be able to co-operate by keeping the arm very still during the dressing, to prevent accidental dislodgement. If there is doubt, assistance may be required.

Equipment/Environment

- The cannula site should be considered as a wound and so should not be exposed unnecessarily or during bed making, dusting, etc.
- Sterile dressing – the type will vary according to local policy, but it should be one that is specially designed for intravenous cannulae.
- If the cannula site requires cleaning, a small dressing pack will be required plus cleansing solution according to local policy.

Nurse

- The hands must be washed and dried thoroughly.
- As there is a risk of direct contact with blood, an apron and gloves should be worn. These should be close-fitting gloves to enable manipulation of self-adhesive dressing and tape.
- Additional protective clothing may be necessary if indicated by the patient's condition (see Chapter 9).

Procedure

1. Ensure that all equipment is within easy reach. Protect the area under the patient's arm with a disposable dressing towel or similar, to collect any spillage.

2. Explain to the patient the importance of remaining still during the procedure, to prevent dislodgement of the cannula.

3. Maintaining asepsis, open the pack and new dressing and pour the cleansing solution (see Aseptic dressing technique, page 258).

4. Put on the sterile gloves, and using the sterile disposal bag as a 'glove' (see page 260), carefully remove the old dressing, taking care not to dislodge the cannula. Assistance may be required to secure the cannula during this procedure.

5. If necessary, clean the cannula site `PFP2`. Inspect the site for signs of phlebitis, infection or extravasation/tissuing (redness, swelling, etc.).

6. Apply the new dressing, taking care not to touch the part that will be directly over the insertion site `PFP3`.

7. If an intravenous infusion is running, secure the tubing of the administration set to prevent pulling and accidental dislodgement of the cannula (Figure 3.7).

Post procedure

Patient	Equipment/Environment	Nurse
• Ensure patient comfort and check understanding regarding the intravenous site.	• Dispose of soiled dressing and other waste appropriately.	• Remove gloves and apron and wash hands. • Document the care and report any abnormalities.

Points for practice

1. The dressing will need changing if it becomes wet, blood-stained or is no longer secure (RCN 2003). If it is clean, dry and secure, most local policies will state that it does not need to be changed until the cannula is removed or re-sited.

2. The site should only require cleaning if there is blood present. If pus or exudate is present, the cannula should be removed.

3. If bandaging is required to protect the cannula site (e.g. a confused patient), it will need to be removed regularly to allow visual observation of the site. A light bandage that does not compress the vein should be used.

REMOVAL OF PERIPHERAL CANNULA

Preparation

Patient	Equipment/Environment	Nurse
• Explain the procedure, to gain consent and co-operation PFP1.	• The cannula site should be considered as a wound and so should not be exposed unnecessarily or during bed making. • Sterile gauze squares. • Small self-adhesive dressing, or tape and sterile gauze. • Yellow clinical waste bag. • Sharps bin.	• The hands must be washed and dried thoroughly. • An apron and gloves should be worn. These should be close-fitting to enable manipulation of adhesive dressings and tape. • Additional protective clothing may be necessary if indicated by the patient's condition (see Chapter 9).

Procedure

1. Put on gloves.
2. Remove the old dressing, leaving the cannula in situ.
3. Fold a piece of gauze three or four times to create an absorbent pad.
4. Place the folded gauze over the cannula insertion site. Gently withdraw the cannula and immediately apply firm pressure over the insertion site.
5. Continue to apply pressure until the bleeding has stopped (about 3 minutes) to prevent haematoma formation.
6. Apply a small dressing, or tape and a piece of sterile gauze, over the site.

Post procedure

Patient	Equipment/Environment	Nurse
• Ensure comfort and advise the patient to report any bleeding or discomfort at the site.	• Discard all waste, including the plastic cannula, into the clinical waste bag.	• Remove gloves and apron and wash hands. • Document removal of cannula and report any abnormalities.

Points for practice

1. Routine replacement of peripheral cannulae every 48–72 hours is generally recommended to prevent phlebitis and catheter colonisation. However, one study found no difference when the cannula was left for 96 hours (Wilson 2006). Refer to your organisation's infection control policy.

References and further reading

Lavery I, Ingram P. (2005) Venepuncture: best practice. *Nursing Standard* **19**(49):55–65.

This is a continuing professional development article that provides guidance on the theory and practice of venepuncture. It includes a useful overview of the anatomy & physiology, choice of sites and special considerations, such as if the patient has had a cerebrovascular accident (stroke). Detailed discussion about prevention of infection and other complications and the technique itself using a syringe and needle and a vacuum system.

Royal College of Nursing. (2003) *Standards for infusion therapy.* RCN, London.

This document provides a comprehensive overview and best practice guidance on all aspects of infusion therapy including: infection control and safety, equipment, site selection, site care and complications.

Snelling P, Duffy L. (2002) Developing self-directed training for intravenous cannulation. *Professional Nurse* **18**:137–142.

This article describes the development of an evidence-based care plan and flexible system of training, using videos and workbooks, that was introduced to help nurses practice cannulation after training. It includes some excellent photographs of the cannulation technique as a step-by-step guide.

Wilson J. (2006) *Infection control in clinical practice.* 3rd edn. Baillière Tindall, Elsevier, Edinburgh.

A comprehensive text that explains basic microbiology, types of organisms and how they are spread. It then provides guidance on infection control practices, preventing wound infections and infections associated with catheters, intravenous cannulae and the respiratory and gastrointestinal systems.

Notes

4

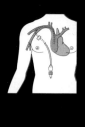

Central venous catheters

CARE OF THE SITE

Preparation

Patient	Equipment/Environment	Nurse
• Explain the procedure, to gain consent and co-operation PFP1. • The patient should be in a recumbent or semi-recumbent position.	• Ensure warmth, privacy and adequate light. • Dressing trolley or clean, flat surface adjacent to the patient. • Sterile dressing pack containing gloves. • Cleansing solution according to local policy (e.g. chlorhexidine in alcohol). • Sterile dressing according to policy/protocol PFP2. • Alcohol hand-rub.	• The hands must be washed and dried thoroughly. • An apron should be worn. • Additional protective clothing may be necessary if indicated by the patient's condition (see Chapter 9).

Procedure

1. Assemble all equipment at the bedside.

2. Ask/assist the patient into a comfortable recumbent or semi-recumbent position and remove clothing as necessary to expose the site PFP3.

3. Open the pack, and using the sterile disposal bag as a 'glove', and taking great care not to dislodge the catheter, remove the old dressing and turn the bag inside out to contain it (see page 260). Place the bag in a convenient position to allow easy access without passing used swabs across the open dressing pack.

4. Put on sterile gloves and, if necessary, clean the site according to local policy and allow it to dry.

5. Apply the new dressing, making sure that the intravenous tubing is secured under the dressing, to prevent pulling on the catheter.

6. Remove gloves.

Post procedure

Patient	Equipment/Environment	Nurse
• Assist the patient as necessary to replace clothing and adopt a comfortable position. • Instruct the patient to report any pain or discomfort at the site.	• Dispose of all waste appropriately.	• Remove apron and wash hands. • Document the dressing change in the nursing records and report any abnormal findings PFP4.

Points for practice

1. The central venous catheter (CVC) insertion site should be inspected at least daily. The dressing will need changing if blood or serous fluid has collected around the catheter, as this greatly increases the infection risk (Wilson 2006).

2. Local policy or protocol will determine the type of dressing to be used. Transparent, moisture-permeable dressings are popular because they are occlusive, allow easy visualisation of the site, and provide secure fixing of the intravenous tubing, thus preventing it pulling on the catheter.

3. A catheter for measurement of the central venous pressure (CVP) will be inserted into the internal or external jugular vein or subclavian vein. Central venous catheters for parenteral nutrition or drug administration (and, therefore, not for CVP measurement) may be inserted into the brachial vein at the antecubital fossa and then advanced until the tip rests in the subclavian vein. This is referred to as a peripherally inserted central catheter (PICC) (Simcock 2001a).

4. CVCs that are no longer required should be removed as soon as possible to reduce the risk of infection (Simcock 2001b)

CVP MEASUREMENT

Preparation

Patient	Equipment/Environment	Nurse
• Explain the procedure, to gain consent and co-operation.	• CVP manometer with 0.9% sodium chloride infusion. CVP measurements cannot be made with any other solution.	• Wash and dry hands thoroughly. Additional protective clothing may be necessary if indicated by the patient's condition (see Chapter 9).
• The patient should be lying flat or in the same position as adopted for previous CVP measurements PFP1.		• Check previous CVP measurements and the position of the patient during these measurements (this should be indicated on the chart).

Procedure

1. With the patient lying flat or in the same position as adopted for previous measurements, level the zero point on the manometer with the patient's heart. A spirit level is incorporated into the manometer arm to ensure accurate levelling (see Figure 4.1).

2. A mark should be made at the mid-axillary line or sternal angle to indicate the level, so that all subsequent readings are made from the same point. This is in line with the right atrium.

3. If necessary, turn off any other infusions that may be running through the central venous catheter.

4. With the three-way tap in position 'A' (Figure 4.1), allow the 0.9% sodium chloride infusion to run rapidly for a few seconds to check that the line is patent PFP2.

5. Stop the infusion by closing the roller clamp. Adjust the three-way tap on the manometer to position 'B', so that the fluid can go up the column. Gradually open the roller clamp to allow fluid to slowly fill the manometer column until 5–10 cm above the previous measurement. Close the roller clamp.

6. Turn the three-way tap to position 'C', so that the line to the infusion bag is closed and the other two lines (to the column and the patient) are open. The fluid in the column will now start to fall, pausing with each respiration, until it equalises with the pressure in the right atrium of the heart. The fluid should continue to rise and fall gently with respiration PFP3. This level, which is measured in centimetres of water (cmH_2O), is the CVP measurement PFP4.

7. Turn the three-way tap back to position 'A', so that the column of fluid is 'off', and reset the infusion to the prescribed rate. Reset any other infusions as appropriate.

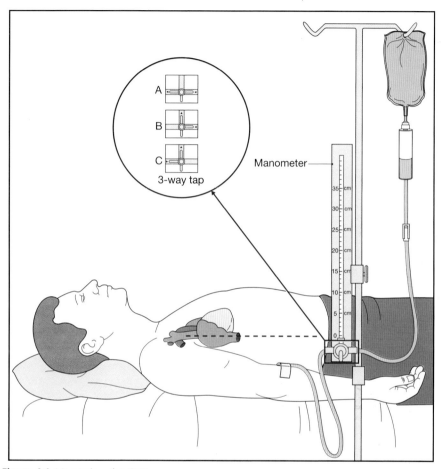

Figure 4.1 Measuring the CVP

Post procedure

Patient	Equipment/Environment	Nurse
• Assist the patient into a comfortable position.	• Ensure all equipment is secured safely and intravenous tubing does not touch the floor.	• Record the CVP measurement on the appropriate chart. If this is the first measurement, also note the position of the patient and the reference point for readings. • Report any abnormalities or changes from previous measurements.

Points for practice

1. The patient needs to be in the same position for all readings to allow comparisons to be made and trends to be observed. If the patient's condition will allow, lying flat will be the most accurate.

2. If the infusion will not run freely, the CVP measurement will not be accurate. Sometimes, asking the patient to turn their head away from the CVP line or applying gentle traction on the line can help by moving the tip of the catheter away from the wall of the blood vessel. If this makes the infusion run freely, perform the same manoeuvre when measuring the CVP.

3. The fluid in the column should rise and fall gently or 'swing' with each respiration because of changes in the pressure within the chest. If the fluid falls but does not swing, it may not be an accurate measurement.

4. The normal range for the CVP is 7–12 cmH$_2$O if measured at the mid axilla, and 0–7 cmH$_2$O if measured at the sternal angle (Naughton 2006). The reading should be interpreted in conjunction with other signs and the trend (i.e. whether it is rising or falling) is often more important than a single measurement.

REMOVAL OF CVC (NON-TUNNELLED)

Preparation

Patient	Equipment/Environment	Nurse
• Explain the procedure, to ensure understanding and co-operation.	• Equipment to perform dressing (page 254).	• Experienced nurses may remove non-tunnelled CVP catheters PFP3. A second nurse may be required to assist during this procedure.
• The patient should be lying flat and slightly head-down if possible PFP1.	• Sterile air-occlusive dressing PFP2.	
	• Sterile scissors and specimen pot (universal type).	• The hands must be washed and dried thoroughly.
• Ensure warmth, dignity and privacy.	• Cleansing solution according to local policy (e.g. povidone iodine).	• An apron should be worn.
	• Stitch cutter and sharps bin.	
	• Alcohol hand-rub or hand washing facilities.	

Procedure

1. Ask/assist the patient to lie flat. Tilt the head of the bed down (about 15°), if the patient's condition will allow. Remove clothing, bedclothes, etc., as necessary to expose the CVP catheter site.

2. Prepare all equipment (see page 258).

3. Turn off the infusion and loosen but do not remove the dressing covering the site.

4. Wash and dry your hands thoroughly or clean them with alcohol hand-rub.

5. Open the dressing pack, and using the waste disposal bag as a 'glove' to protect your hand, remove the dressing and turn the bag inside out to contain it (see page 260). Place the bag in a convenient position to allow easy access.

6. Put on the sterile gloves provided in the dressing pack, and using a gauze swab and cleansing solution, clean around the insertion site PFP4.

7. Use the stitch cutter to cut the stitch holding the catheter in place and make sure it is free of the skin.

8. Maintaining sterility, open the specimen pot and place it in an accessible position.

9. Fold a gauze square two or three times to create an absorbent pad. Holding this in your non-dominant hand, place it over the insertion site, ready to press immediately the catheter is withdrawn.

10. Ask the patient to hold their breath during removal of the catheter. Withdraw the catheter by pulling in a firm, steady movement and press firmly

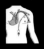

with the gauze pad for several minutes to prevent bleeding and air embolus PFP1.

11. Ask an assistant to place the tip of the catheter in the specimen pot, and using sterile scissors, cut off the tip (about 5 cm) and allow it to fall into the container. Replace the lid PFP5.

12. Once the bleeding has stopped, apply the sterile air-occlusive dressing to the site.

13. Remove gloves.

Post procedure

Patient	Equipment/Environment	Nurse
• Return the bed to the horizontal position and ask the patient to remain supine for 15–30 minutes following removal.	• Dispose of all clinical waste and sharps appropriately.	• Wash and dry hands thoroughly. • Label the specimen container, and with the appropriate request form, send for bacteriological examination. • Document CVP removal in the nursing records

Points for practice

1. There is a significant risk of air embolism during and after the removal of a CVP catheter (Menim et al 1992). Placing the patient in a supine, head-down position reduces this by increasing the intrathoracic pressure, making it less likely for air to be drawn in during inspiration. Forceful inspiration, e.g. following a cough, may facilitate entry of air (Woodrow 2002).

2. An air-occlusive dressing must be used to reduce the risk of air entry leading to air embolus following removal of the catheter (RCN 2003).

3. Local policy may dictate that only nurses who have undergone additional training may remove CVP catheters. Tunnelled catheters must be removed by medical staff and often require surgical removal.

4. The site must be cleaned before removal of the catheter, to prevent contamination of the tip during withdrawal. This would lead to an inaccurate bacteriological assessment (see below).

5. Trust protocol may require the tip of the catheter to be sent for bacterial examination following removal if catheter-related sepsis is suspected (RCN 2003). If no assistance is available, place the catheter on the trolley so that the tip is resting on a corner of the sterile field, to prevent contamination. Once the dressing is securely in place, cut the tip off as described.

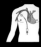

CARE OF LONG-TERM CVCs

Principles

Hickman and Groshong lines are types of central venous catheters made of special hypoallergenic material that allow them to remain in situ for many months. They are often used for patients who require regular, but intermittent, intravenous therapy, such as those receiving chemotherapy or total parenteral nutrition (TPN). As with all central venous catheters, there is a high risk of infection, especially with patients who are immunosuppressed and/or receiving chemotherapy and, therefore, asepsis is vital. In order to reduce the risk of infection, long-term catheters are tunnelled under the skin (Figure 4.2). This means that the insertion site through the skin, which is very vulnerable to infection, is well away from the point of entry into the blood vessel, thus reducing the risk of septicaemia (Simcock 2001b). Most tunnelled CVCs have a dacron 'cuff' situated approximately 1.5 cm from the exit site (Figure 4.2). As the patient's tissues grow around the cuff it secures the CVC in place and acts as a barrier to infection (Gabriel 2001).

Care of the site

Care of long-term catheters is often undertaken at home by patients or carers or by the district nurse. The dressing over the cannula site should be changed twice weekly until the tissue around the Dacron cuff has become fibrosed. Long-term care varies considerably from hospital to hospital, but covering the site is not usually necessary once the site has healed, except when there is a risk of it getting wet, e.g. in the shower.

Immersion of the site is not recommended, but splashing, as in the shower, is usually no problem. Bathing in a public pool and water sports are not

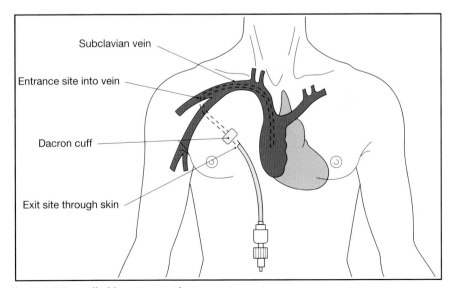

Figure 4.2 Tunnelled long-term catheter

recommended because of the risk of infection from the water. In order to remain patent, the catheter must be flushed at regular intervals to prevent clotting. Most hospitals recommend the use of heparinised saline two to three times per week, but recommended practices vary in both frequency and the solution used.

Care of implantable ports

Implantable ports are designed for long-term intermittent venous access. They are surgically implanted under the skin of the chest wall or sometimes on the arm. It is sutured to the underlying muscle to anchor it in place. The device may have one or two ports, each of which is attached to a single lumen catheter, which is inserted into the vein. Once the wound has healed the port is accessed by insertion of a needle through the skin and through the injectable membrane of the device. Once the infusion or drug has been administered that needle is removed and the port seals off, thus reducing the risk of infection. It is almost invisible under the skin and so is more discreet that a tunnelled device, but it does require the patient to have regular needles through the skin.

Total parenteral nutrition

Total parenteral nutrition (TPN) is most commonly administered via a central venous catheter, which because of the irritant nature of the high dextrose solution, is the route of choice. Tunnelled CVP catheters are recommended for TPN; however, administration via a peripheral line is used in some situations. The administration set being used for TPN must be changed every 24 hours with each new bag. The bags of feed must be stored in a designated refrigerator and removed 2 hours prior to administration (1 hour may be sufficient in hot weather). If there are no lipids in the bag, it must be covered to prevent degradation of the vitamins by exposure to light.

The line must be flushed with 0.9% sodium chloride containing heparin before commencing and after completion of a feed. The CVP catheter being used for TPN must not be used for measurement or drug administration because any interruption in the closed system increases the risk of infection. There is also a high risk of incompatibility with medicines.

References and further reading

Dougherty L, Lamb J. (1999) *Intravenous therapy in nursing practice*. Churchill Livingstone, London.

This is a comprehensive UK text book that addresses all aspects of intravenous therapy in a variety of care settings. It also includes a chapter on intravenous therapy in children. The second edition is due to be published in December 2007.

Gabriel L. (2001) PICC securement: minimising potential complications. *Nursing Standard* **15**(43):42–44.

This article discusses the uses and advantages of peripherally inserted central catheters (PICC), methods of securement and prevention of complications.

Hamilton H. (2004) Central venous catheters: choosing the most appropriate access route. *British Journal of Nursing* **13**(14):862–870.

A comprehensive examination of the evidence to support the choice of insertion site for CVCs and the attendant risks and complications.

Ingram P, Sinclair L, Edwards T. (2006) The safe removal of central venous catheters. *Nursing Standard* **20**(49):42–46.

An excellent article that provides detailed guidelines for the removal of CVCs with supporting rationale. It has a particular focus on reducing the risk of air embolus.

Jones CA. (2006) Central venous catheter infection in adults in acute hospital settings. *British Journal of Nursing* **15**(7):364–368.

This article presents a literature review of recent research on measures used to reduce CVC-related infections, which is then compared to current best practice. The author concludes that the evidence mainly backs up current practice but argues that skin disinfection could be improved and stressed the importance of good hand hygiene and education programmes.

Mennim P, Coyle C, Taylor J. (1992) Venous air embolism associated with removal of central venous catheter. *British Medical Journal* **305**:171–172.

Although this paper is now over 15 years old, it still contains excellent advice about the risks of air embolus during removal of CVP and ways to minimise that risk.

Pratt R. (2001) Preventing infections associated with central venous catheters. *Nursing Times* **97**(15):36–39.

Evidence-based guidelines that focus on the prevention of bloodstream infections. It includes the choice of type of CVC and the risks associated with each.

Royal College of Nursing. (2003) *Standards for infusion therapy*. RCN, London.

This document provides a comprehensive overview and best practice guidance on all aspects of infusion therapy and CVCs including: infection control and safety, equipment, site selection, site care and complications and removal of CVC.

Simcock L. (2001a) The use of central venous catheters for IV therapy. *Nursing Times* **97** (18):34–35.

This article provides a useful overview of the types of central venous catheters available: tunnelled, non-tunnelled, peripherally inserted and implantable ports, with diagrams of each.

Simcock L. (2001b) Central venous catheters: some common clinical questions. *Nursing Times* **97**(19):34–35.

This article contains some useful answers to practical questions such as 'Do I need to wear sterile gloves when changing the dressing?' 'How often should it be flushed?' and 'How often should I change the dressing?'. It provides a useful table that compares the advantages and disadvantages of the different types of dressings available.

Woodrow P. (2002) Central venous catheters and central venous pressure. *Nursing Standard* **16**(26):45–52.

This is a continuing professional development article that addresses all aspects of CVC management and CVP measurement. This includes: the rationale for CVC insertion, technique for reading the CVP, reasons for and significance of abnormal readings, complications and technique for removal of CVC.

Wilson J. (2006) *Infection control in clinical practice*. 3rd edn. Baillière Tindall, Elsevier, Edinburgh.

A comprehensive text that explains basic microbiology, types of organisms and how they are spread. It then provides guidance on infection control practices, preventing wound infections and infections associated with catheters, intravenous cannulae and the respiratory and gastrointestinal systems.

5

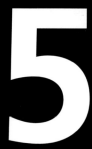

Blood transfusion

CHECKING COMPATIBILITY

Principles

- It is vital that blood for transfusion is checked carefully to ensure that the correct blood is administered to the correct patient. Fatal consequences can ensue if the incorrect blood is given.

- Adverse reactions most commonly occur within 10–15 minutes of commencing transfusion and so it is vital that nurses continually observe the patient during this time. The frequency of observations after that time will vary according to local policy but according to the British Committee for Standards in Haematology (BCSH 1999) further observations need only be taken if the patient becomes unwell or shows signs of a transfusion reaction. Therefore, regular visual observation throughout the transfusion is vital. For this reason it is recommended that blood transfusions are only given at night when absolutely necessary as staffing levels are lower and there may a reluctance to disturb sleeping patients to perform observations (Stevenson 2007).

- Until relatively recently, blood was always checked by two nurses, one of whom had to be a registered nurse, and many local policies require this. However, guidance from the British Committee for Standards in Haematology (BCSH 1999) now suggests that it may be safer for one registered nurse to carry out the checking procedure to avoid the risk of each relying on each other to check thoroughly. Whatever the policy, **it is vital that all checking is carried out at the bedside**.

- All patients receiving a blood transfusion must wear an identification name band.

Storage of blood

- Blood must be stored in a special refrigerator at 2–6°C to prevent contaminants reproducing. It **must not** be kept in a ward refrigerator.

- Blood for transfusion should be collected from the blood transfusion department or special refrigerator no longer than 30 minutes before it is required. This is because pathogens grow extremely quickly in blood at room temperature. If the transfusion has not commenced within this time, the blood bank must be informed and the blood may need to be discarded (RCN 2004).

- If the blood is stored in a special 'blood carrier' this time may be extended (see local policy).

Blood bag

- The bag should be checked to ensure that it is not leaking or wet and that there is no turbidity or discoloration.

- The bag must have a compatibility label attached (Figure 5.1).

- Drugs must never be added to blood.

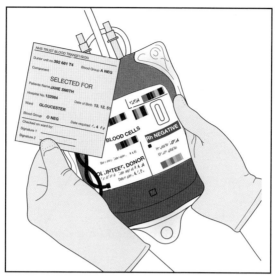

Figure 5.1 Blood bag with compatibility label

- Blood must never be warmed by placing it in hot water or in a microwave. Direct heat will cause blood to haemolyse (Bradbury & Cruickshank 2000). If warming is required, a blood warmer should be used (see below and page 106).

Administration

- A special blood administration set that incorporates a filter chamber must be used. An additional in-line filter may be required where multiple units of blood are to be administered. Refer to local policy.

- There is no evidence that warming the blood is beneficial if it is administered slowly, but if rapid transfusion of large volumes is required (>50 ml/kg/hour) or blood is being administered via a central venous catheter, a blood warmer should be used (Bradbury & Cruickshank 2000). Blood must **never** be warmed by placing into hot water, a microwave or on a radiator (BCSH 1999).

- Some infusion pumps may damage blood cells and should only be used if the manufacturer's instructions specifically state that they are safe to use for that purpose.

Documentation

- All documentation must be thoroughly checked during the checking process; do not rely solely on the patient's name band to confirm the name and hospital number; the medical case notes, the blood transfusion compatibility report form, the compatibility label and the prescription chart must also be checked (see checking procedure below).

Blood transfusion checking procedure

1. **Check the patient's identity**
   - All checking must take place at the bedside.
   - Where possible, positively identify patients by asking them to state their full name and date of birth. Check that these match the name band.

2. **Check the patient's surname, first names, sex, date of birth, hospital number, blood group and rhesus factor on:**
   - Patient's name band.
   - Blood transfusion compatibility report form.
   - Compatibility label attached to the bag.
   - Medical case notes.
   - Intravenous (IV) fluid prescription chart.

3. **Check the expiry date of the unit of blood (and time if applicable, e.g. platelets) on:**
   - Compatibility label on the bag.
   - Blood bag.

4. **Check the blood group and unit number on:**
   - Blood transfusion compatibility report form.
   - Compatibility label on the bag.

5. **Check any special requirements**
   - The unit of blood must comply with the prescription chart (e.g. gamma irradiated).

6. **Record the unit number of the blood on:**
   - The intravenous (IV) fluid prescription chart.

7. **Record the date and time and signature of the nurse(s) on:**
   - Blood transfusion compatibility report form.
   - Compatibility label.
   - Intravenous (IV) fluid prescription chart.

If any discrepancies are noted, the blood must not be transfused, the blood bank must be informed, and the blood and blood transfusion compatibility form returned.

CARE AND MANAGEMENT OF A TRANSFUSION

Preparation

Patient	Equipment/Environment	Nurse
• Explain the procedure, to gain consent and co-operation PFP1.	• Blood administration set PFP2.	• Wash and dry hands thoroughly.
• The patient must be wearing a name band.	• Clinical thermometer and watch.	• Gloves and an apron should be worn.
• Advise the patient not to leave the ward during the transfusion (in many instances patients will be confined to bed).	• Sphygmomanometer and stethoscope.	
• Unconscious patients require very close monitoring.	• Observation chart (temperature, pulse, respiration and blood pressure).	
	• Fluid balance chart.	
	• Intravenous prescription chart.	
	• Intravenous adrenaline (epinephrine) and chlorpheniramine should be available on the ward (in case of allergic reactions).	

Procedure

1. At the bedside, check the blood as described on page 100. Blood must be checked by a registered nurse, before transfusion. Some local policies will require two nurses to check (see page 100).

2. Prepare the infusion as described on page 72.

3. Record baseline observations of temperature, pulse, respiration and blood pressure immediately prior to commencement of the transfusion.

4. Calculate the rate of infusion and set the infusion to the required rate (see page 78) PFP3.

5. Observe the patient continuously for the first 15 minutes as this is when a reaction is most likely to occur. Record the temperature, pulse, respiration and blood pressure again 15 minutes after commencement of the transfusion. These observations should be repeated at regular intervals throughout the transfusion according to local policy PFP4 and again at the end of the transfusion.

6. Observe the urine output for volume and colour throughout the transfusion PFP5.

7. Observe for and encourage the patient to report any of the following (Shamash 2002) PFP6:

Allergic reaction/anaphylaxis (allergic reaction to 'foreign' plasma proteins):
- Wheezing and shortness of breath
- Hypotension
- A rash on the chest or abdomen
- Oedema of the eyes or face
- Laryngeal swelling

Febrile reaction (reaction of the patient's antibodies to donor leucocytes):
- Pyrexia
- Feeling hot and flushed or shivering
- Rigors

Haemolytic reaction (most serious reaction, due to transfusion of incompatible blood):
- Chest or abdominal pain, or pain in the extremities
- Lumbar or loin pain
- Oliguria
- Hypotension and shock

Circulatory overload (more common in elderly especially those with heart failure):
- Rising pulse and respiration rates
- Dyspnoea or 'bubbly' respiration and frothy sputum
- Hypotension.

8. **The transfusion should be stopped and medical staff informed if:**
   - there is a rise in temperature of greater than 1°C
   - there is a significant rise or fall in blood pressure
   - there is a significant rise in pulse rate
   - any of the above reactions occur.

9. If the transfusion continues for more than 12 hours, the administration set should be changed every 12 hours to prevent bacterial growth.

10. The blood transfusion compatibility form must be readily available throughout the transfusion.

Post procedure

Patient	Equipment/Environment	Nurse
• Ensure the patient is comfortable. • Instruct the patient to observe for and report any reaction or complications.	• Replace equipment and discard waste appropriately. • The empty blood bags should be dealt with according to local policy **PFP7**. • Change the administration set every 12 hours during the transfusion and at the end of the transfusion if an intravenous infusion is to follow.	• Document the blood transfusion in the nursing records. • Secure the blood transfusion compatibility report form in the medical notes. • Report any abnormalities or complications.

Points for practice

1. Written consent is not usually required but patients must be fully informed (RCN 2003). Some patients have a cultural and religious objection to blood transfusion, e.g. Jehovah's Witnesses, and their wishes must be respected (McInroy 2005).

2. A special administration set must be used for blood transfusions. This has an additional chamber above the drip chamber, which contains a filter. This filters out debris (platelets and white cells) (see Figure 3.4B, page 72). Platelet administration requires a special administration set with no filter. Platelets must be administered rapidly (20–30 minutes) as soon as they are available.

3. Electronic infusion pumps may damage blood cells and must only be used if the manufacturer's instructions specifically state that they can be used to administer blood (BCSH 1999).

4. Observations during blood transfusion should be clearly dated and recorded separately from routine observations in case retrieval at a later date is necessary (BCSH 1999). Trust policies regarding the frequency of the observations required during blood transfusion may vary, but most suggest that the temperature, pulse, respiration rate and blood pressure should be recorded before the start of the transfusion, 15 minutes after commencement, and again at the end of the transfusion. Each unit of blood should be regarded as a new transfusion. The first 15 minutes of a transfusion is the period when severe reactions most commonly occur (Bradbury & Cruickshank 2000).

5. The urine output should be monitored for haemoglobinuria or oliguria, which are signs of an acute haemolytic transfusion reaction.

6. If an adverse reaction occurs, the transfusion must be stopped immediately and the medical staff informed. The administration set should be changed and venous access maintained by an infusion of 0.9% sodium chloride. The patient's temperature, pulse, respiration rate and blood pressure, and the colour and volume of urine should be monitored (RCN 2003).

7. Ideally used blood bags are kept for at least 2 days following transfusion in case there is a delayed reaction to the blood (BCSH 1999). The procedure for storage and ultimate disposal of blood bags will vary from hospital to hospital.

USE OF BLOOD FILTERS AND BLOOD WARMERS

Blood filters

- A blood administration set that includes a 170 mm filter chamber is all that is required for most blood transfusions.

- Some patients who are receiving multiple blood transfusions or who have had febrile reactions in response to previous transfusions may require an additional filter. These are fine-mesh filters that are placed between the blood bag and the administration set in order to remove microaggregates (e.g. fibrin and clots) formed during storage. The same filter can be used for up to four units of blood. If a filter is required it is usually supplied with the blood when collected from the blood transfusion department.

Blood warmers

- When rapid transfusion or transfusion via a CVP line is necessary, blood may be warmed during administration using a blood warmer. Blood must never be warmed by heating the bag in hot water, on a radiator or in a microwave, as direct heat can cause blood to haemolyse. The design of blood warmers will vary, but most incorporate a 'zig-zag' tube or coil through which the blood passes over a heater element and is warmed before reaching the patient.

References and further reading

Bradbury M, Cruickshank J. (2000) Blood transfusion: crucial steps in maintaining safe practice. *British Journal of Nursing* **9**(3):134–138.

This article considers nurses' responsibilities in relation to safe administration of blood and provides evidence-based guidelines using the mnemonic PACK: Patient & Pre-transfusion checks; Asepsis & Apparatus; Checking & Clerical procedures; Keeping vigilant and Keeping accurate records.

British Committee for Standards in Haematology (BCSH). (1999) The administration of blood and blood products and the management of transfused patients. *Transfusion Medicine* **9**:227–238.

This provides detailed guidelines on all aspects of blood transfusion from collection of blood samples for cross-matching to the type and frequency of observations during transfusion. It includes an excellent summary of the possible complications of blood transfusion, their causes and when they are most likely to occur. This is the most recent available guidance from BCSH but it is worth checking their website and the SHOT and Department of Health websites (see below) regularly for updates.

McInroy A. (2005) Blood transfusion and Jehovah's Witnesses: the legal and ethical issues. *British Journal of Nursing* **14**(5):270–274.

An interesting article that examines the legal and ethical issues surrounding a patient's right to refuse blood transfusion and what type of blood products might be acceptable.

Royal College of Nursing. (2004) Right blood, right patient, right time. *Guidelines for the safe administration of blood and blood products*. RCN, London.

This is available from the RCN website *www.rcn.org.uk* and provides comprehensive evidence-based guidance on all aspects of blood transfusion from obtaining the blood sample for cross-matching to patient monitoring during transfusion.

Shamesh J. (2002) Blood counts. *Nursing Times* **98**(45):23–26.

An interesting article that provides some statistics and the history of blood transfusions. It discusses all aspects from blood donation to transfusion observations and provides a nice overview of the most common complications. Also has a good list of useful contacts and resources.

Stevenson T. (2007) The safe administration of blood transfusions at night. *Nursing Times* **103**(5):33–34.

This paper reports an audit of blood transfusions at night in a district general hospital and found that two-thirds could have safely been delayed until morning. They suggest that, because of the greater risk of error and delayed detection of any reaction, nurses should challenge the need for transfusions at night and suggest that Trust protocols should also reflect this. They also stress that if transfusion at night is necessary greater vigilance is required to ensure patient safety.

Websites

British Committee for Standards in Haematology. www.bcshguidelines.com

Department of Health Better blood transfusions. www.doh.gov.uk/blood

SHOT (serious hazards of transfusion). www.shotuk.org

Notes

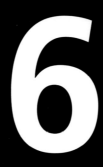
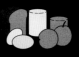

6

Nutrition and hydration

NUTRITIONAL ASSESSMENT

Principles

Good nutrition is essential not only to promote health and well-being, but also to aid recovery from trauma, surgery or disease. Yet there is growing evidence that malnutrition is common among hospital patients. Malnutrition is referred to in the Nutrition Support Clinical Guideline as a state in which a deficiency of nutrients causes measurable adverse effects on body function and/or clinical outcome (NICE 2006). Although malnutrition or 'bad nutrition' associated with over-eating is also an important issue for nurses undertaking nutritional assessment, the focus of much of the literature has been on under-nutrition. Poor nutritional status is known to be associated with delayed recovery and adverse outcomes of illness and injury (Holmes 2003). Nurses have an important role to play in the prevention of malnutrition. An important part of their role is to identify those at risk of malnutrition and plan care to meet their needs. In addition they have a role in ensuring those who are initially well-nourished do not become malnourished whilst in hospital. Appropriate and ongoing nutritional assessment is vital.

Nutritional assessment tools

Although most hospitals have developed a tool to assist in nutritional assessment and the identification of those at risk, the National Institute of Clinical Excellence (NICE 2006) recommend use of the validated Malnutrition Universal Screening Tool (MUST). Its components consist of the following:

1. Body Mass Index
2. Recent unplanned weight loss
3. Subjective criteria (such as those outlined below)
4. Once risk is established, use local guidelines and/or policies to develop appropriate care plans.

Body Mass Index (BMI) is a tool for use with patients over 18 years of age and enables determination of whether the patient has a normal weight, is underweight or overweight. However, on its own it is not a good indicator of nutritional risk; it needs to be used in conjunction with other measures. BMI is calculated by dividing the weight in kilograms (kg) by the height in metres squared (see below). If the patient is unable to stand, arm span can be used instead of height. This is measured by extending both arms sideways from the body at shoulder height and measuring the distance between the tips of the middle fingers. A BMI of 20–24.9 indicates an average or desirable weight. A BMI of greater than 30 is classified as obese and greater than 40 as grossly obese. Patients with a BMI of less than 20 may show signs of under-nutrition. It is important to note, however, that patients who are overweight or obese can also be malnourished.

$$\text{BMI} = \frac{\text{weight in kg}}{(\text{height in metres})^2} = \frac{60}{1.69 \times 1.69} = 20.01$$

In addition to the BMI, most nutritional assessment tools will incorporate consideration of the following factors, which are known to increase the risk of malnutrition (Holmes 2003, Holmes 2006, NICE 2006):

- Age – older adults are vulnerable to under-nutrition and its incidence rises with age irrespective of illness. A decline in lean body mass (LBM) reduces basal metabolic rate by 10–15% or more after 50 years of age. Loss of LBM enhances morbidity and mortality and impacts on cardiac, respiratory and muscle function as well as reducing body temperature (hypothermia) and increasing the risk of falls and subsequent injury.

- Mental condition – any deterioration in mental state or conscious level is likely to affect the patient's desire and ability to eat and drink independently and so will increase the risk of malnutrition. This includes patients who may be depressed, lethargic or apathetic.

- Weight – it is important to note whether there has been any recent weight loss, particularly if it is unintentional. This may be apparent from loose-fitting clothes, rings or dentures. Patients who appear thin or emaciated are at an increased risk of malnutrition. Less than 5% weight loss in 6 months is not significant. Between 5–9% is only significant if the patient is already malnourished. Between 10–20% is clinically significant and requires intervention, and more than 20% weight loss may require long-term support.

- Appetite – patients who are able to maintain their usual appetite and eating habits are less likely to be at risk than those who have a poor appetite or refuse meals and drinks. It is important to check whether the patient has altered their eating habits recently.

- Functioning of the gastrointestinal tract – the presence of diarrhoea or constipation is likely to affect the desire to eat and drink and may also lead to malabsorption. Nausea and vomiting are also likely to result in a reduced nutritional intake. Patients who are unable to take oral food or fluids following surgery involving the gastrointestinal tract or who have conditions that affect it, such as intestinal obstruction, will be at high risk.

- Skin and pressure ulcers – dry and scaling skin may be an indication of dehydration and possibly related malnourishment. The existence of pressure ulcers is significant and is often included on nutritional assessment tools. Pressure ulcers are often associated with poor nutrition and healing pressure ulcers requires increased nutritional intake.

- Dexterity – it is important to assess whether patients have the manual dexterity to feed themselves.

- Other factors – a number of conditions will affect the ability to eat and so will increase the risk of developing malnutrition. These include:
  - neurological conditions, especially those affecting co-ordination or mental state
  - difficulty swallowing (e.g. after stroke) and malabsorption
  - surgery or major trauma

- malignant disease and chronic conditions, such as chronic obstructive pulmonary disease
- reduced mobility or confinement to bed
- bereavement, depression or other mental ill health.

Most nutritional assessment tools involve a scoring system that allocates a score for each of the possible contributing factors. The total score will indicate whether the patient is at risk; appropriate measures can then be taken. Whether a high score indicates a high or a low risk will vary between different assessment tools. Patients identified as high risk should be referred to a dietician and nutritional support should be considered for those who are malnourished or at risk of becoming malnourished (NICE 2006). Patients must be assessed within 24 hours of admission. The frequency of further assessments should be determined by the result of the initial assessment. For example, if a patient is well nourished on admission to hospital then weekly reassessment is adequate. However, if the nutritional assessment score indicates at-risk then reassessment may need to be within 48 hours.

Nutritional support

The NICE (2006) guidelines state that oral, enteral or parenteral nutritional support, either alone or combined, should be considered for people who are malnourished or at risk of malnourishment. They define malnourished as:

- a body mass index (BMI) of less than 18.5 kg/m^2
- unintentional weight loss greater than 10% within the last 3–6 months
- a BMI of less than 20 kg/m^2 and unintentional weight loss greater than 5% within the last 3–6 months.

Risk of malnutrition is defined as:

- having eaten little or nothing for more than 5 days and/or likely to be eating little or nothing in the next 5 days or longer
- where there is an increased nutritional need, where the capacity for absorption is reduced, or where there is a high nutrient loss.

FEEDING ADULTS

Preparation

Patient	Equipment/Environment	Nurse
• Establish what the patient would like to eat and drink and whether there are any dietary restrictions.	• Remove any offensive materials from the patient's table/eating area, e.g. sputum pot, urinals, etc.	• Wash and dry hands thoroughly.
• Ensure the patient is comfortable, i.e. has an empty bladder, clean hands, clean mouth and, if applicable, clean dentures.	• Clear a space for the tray. • Position a chair beside the bed for the nurse. • Napkin or paper towel.	• Additional protective clothing may be necessary if indicated by the patient's condition (see Chapter 9).
• Ask/assist the patient to sit upright if their condition allows.		• Put on apron (appropriate colour if applicable) PFP1.
• Check the patient is able to swallow, to prevent choking and aspiration into the lungs.		

Procedure

1. Aim to make the mealtime a pleasant experience for the patient.
2. Obtain the correct food and drink, cutlery and napkin.
3. Set the meal out in a pleasing manner to tempt the appetite.
4. Take the tray to the bedside, and if the patient is unable to see the food, describe the meal PFP2.
5. Cut up the food if necessary.
6. Protect the patient's clothing with a napkin or paper towel.
7. Sit down so that a more relaxed approach is conveyed to the patient (Figure 6.1). Encourage/support the patient to feed themselves if at all possible, using special cutlery if necessary PFP3.
8. Adjust the speed and manner in which food/drink is offered according to the patient's needs/wishes. It should not be hurried PFP4.
9. Allow the patient time to chew and swallow the food before presenting the next mouthful. Adjust the size of the mouthful to suit the patient.
10. Avoid asking questions while the patient is eating.
11. Respect the patient's dignity and use the napkin to remove dribbles of food or drink that may run down the chin.
12. When giving a drink, tip the cup/glass very gently so that the flow is controlled. Care should be taken with hot drinks, particularly if using a polystyrene cup, as it is difficult to judge the temperature of the liquid inside.

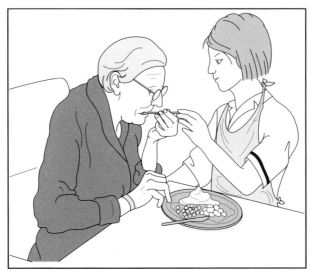

Figure 6.1 Feeding the patient

13. Encourage the patient to eat and drink if necessary, but do not press patients once they have indicated that they have had sufficient. Small amounts taken more frequently may be more successful.

Post procedure

Patient	Equipment/Environment	Nurse
• Assist the patient to meet hygiene needs (mouth, teeth and hands) as necessary.	• Remove unwanted food, crockery and cutlery. • Wipe up any spillages on the table or locker. • Restore the patient's environment, i.e. put a glass of water and the patient's belongings back within easy reach.	• Remove apron and wash hands. • Complete relevant documentation, e.g. fluid balance and/or food chart. • Report any abnormal occurrences, e.g. vomiting, food refusal.

Points for practice

1. In some hospitals, different-coloured aprons are used for activities, such as serving meals, washing patients and doing dressings.
2. If supervising the patient rather than feeding them, place all food and drink within easy reach of the patient. If the patient is visually impaired, 'clock' instructions may help them locate different foods, e.g. meat is at 12 o'clock, potatoes are at 5 o'clock, etc.

3. If the patient is only able to use one hand, a plate guard and non-slip mat may help. If they are unable to grip ordinary cutlery, large-handled cutlery can usually be obtained from the Occupational Therapy department.

4. Always check any particular cultural practices related to eating and drinking. For example, where possible, a Muslim patient should be fed with the right hand as the left hand is considered 'unclean'.

NAUSEA AND VOMITING

Preparation

Patient	Equipment/Environment	Nurse
• Respond promptly to calls for assistance.	• Draw screens if time permits, to ensure privacy.	• Put on apron and gloves (if time).
	• Provide vomit bowl (usually disposable).	• Additional protective clothing may be necessary if indicated by the patient's condition (see Chapter 9).
	• Provide tissues or paper towels.	

Procedure

1. If possible, remove the patient's dentures (where applicable) and store them safely.

2. Ask/assist the patient to sit forward, or if lying down or semi-conscious, place in the lateral position to reduce the risk of aspiration into the lungs.

3. Support the patient's forehead.

4. Encourage the patient to breathe more deeply if possible.

5. Provide tissues and promote comfort and dignity by wiping the patient's mouth if the patient is too weak or distressed to do this unaided.

6. Never leave the patient without a vomit bowl – get a clean one before removing the used one, even if the patient feels the episode has passed.

Post procedure

Patient	Equipment/Environment	Nurse
• Offer a mouthwash or perform mouth care if the patient is too weak.	• Cover the vomit bowl before removing it from the bedside.	• Document the vomiting episode, making a note of nausea, frequency, amount and whether related to food **PFP4**.
• Offer the patient a bowl for face and hand washing.	• Identify the type of vomit and measure the amount **PFP2**.	• Report if vomiting is a new occurrence or if the vomiting has altered in any way.
• If appropriate, administer anti-emetic drugs as prescribed and monitor the effect **PFP1**.	• Save the vomit for inspection if necessary (e.g. haematemesis) **PFP3**.	• Ascertain the cause of vomiting if possible, and take appropriate action.

Points for practice

1. Post-operative nausea and vomiting causes distress and suffering for many surgical patients. The prophylactic administration of prescribed anti-emetic medication can greatly reduce this (Thomas 1999).

2. The vomit may contain undigested food or be watery (gastric juices only) or a green/brown fluid (indicates presence of bile). If the vomit is brown and foul (faecal) smelling, this may indicate that there is an obstruction in the large intestine.

3. The term haematemesis means blood in the vomit. If this is bright red, it indicates fresh blood from the stomach or upper gastrointestinal tract; if it is dark brown and 'coffee ground' in appearance, this is older blood that has been partially digested.

4. Note the amount, frequency, whether accompanied by pain or nausea and whether associated with any medication (e.g. analgesic), surgery, type of food or other cause. Also note whether it is projectile vomit (vomit that is emitted with force).

SUBCUTANEOUS FLUIDS (HYPERDERMOCLYSIS)

Preparation

Patient	Equipment/Environment	Nurse
• Explain the procedure, to gain consent and co-operation.	• Prescribed fluid and additive (if applicable) **PFP2**.	• Wash and dry hands thoroughly and put on gloves.
• Patients receiving subcutaneous fluids are often older adults and are sometimes confused. A second nurse may be required to comfort the patient **PFP1**.	• Standard administration set. • Peripheral plastic cannula (e.g. Insyte-w 24G – 0.7 × 19 mm) or 'butterfly'-type intravenous cannula (21G) **PFP3**. • Transparent occlusive dressing (approximately 10 cm × 10 cm).	• Only registered nurses may insert the cannula and subcutaneous infusions must be checked by a registered nurse.

Procedure

1. Check the prescribed fluid and prime the administration set to expel all air (see page 72) **PFP4**.

2. At the bedside, ask/assist the patient to move into a suitable position to allow access to the site **PFP5**. Check the patient's name band against the prescription.

3. Clean the skin with an alcohol-impregnated swab and allow it to dry.

4. Maintaining asepsis, remove the protective cover from the cannula and hold it with the bevelled edge facing upwards. Pinch the skin up slightly and insert the needle into the subcutaneous tissue at an angle of 45° (Figure 6.2). If blood appears in the tubing, withdraw the cannula and repeat the process at another site using a new cannula.

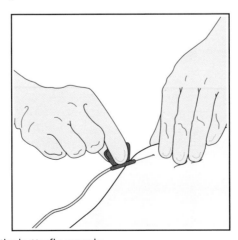

Figure 6.2 Inserting the butterfly cannula

5. Cover the area with the transparent dressing.

6. Set the infusion to the prescribed rate (see page 78).

Post procedure

Patient	Equipment/Environment	Nurse
• Ensure the patient is comfortable.	• Dispose of all clinical waste appropriately.	• Document the subcutaneous infusion in the nursing records.
• Observe the cannula site for redness, swelling or discomfort.		• Record/monitor fluid balance according to local policy.
• Change the infusion site regularly, according to local policy **PFP6**.		

Points for practice

1. Subcutaneous fluids are used most commonly for older adults with dehydration where there is no indication for intravenous fluids. Other palliative benefits have been reported in patients who have constipation or compromised tissue viability or those who have difficulties with oral intake, which makes them prone to dehydration (Barton et al 2004).

2. Dextrose saline or 0.9% sodium chloride are the solutions most commonly administered subcutaneously. An enzyme (hyaluronidase), which causes more rapid diffusion of the fluid by reducing normal interstitial barriers, may be prescribed. It may be injected into the site via the cannula prior to commencement of the infusion, or added to the infusion bag. However, there is little clinical evidence to support its use (Barton et al 2004, Moriarty & Hudson 2001).

3. This may vary according to local policy or practice guidelines as the use of Teflon or Vailon needles instead of steel winged infusion devices has been associated with fewer complications and reduces the need for frequent needle changes (Ross et al 2002).

4. In most cases, all subcutaneous fluids must be checked by a registered nurse, although this may vary according to local policy. In some Trusts, two nurses are required to check intravenous and subcutaneous fluids.

5. Any site with sufficient subcutaneous tissue may be used, but oedematous areas must be avoided. The nurse should consider patient comfort, mobility, ease of access and skin condition when choosing the site. The abdomen and thighs are commonly used, although the areas over the scapula and anterior chest wall are ideal.

6. Ideally the infusion site should be changed after 2 l of fluid or every 24 hours, although every 48 hours has been suggested as adequate (Mansfield 1998). The giving set should be changed at least every 72 hours (RCN 2003).

NASOGASTRIC TUBE INSERTION

Preparation

Patient	Equipment/Environment	Nurse
• Explain the procedure, to gain consent and co-operation.	• Prepare space at the bedside.	• Wash and dry hands thoroughly.
• Draw screens to ensure privacy.	• Nasogastric tube of appropriate size and type (e.g. Ryles type, fine bore) PFP2.	• Put on apron and gloves.
• Ensure the patient is comfortable – sitting upright if possible, with the head neither tilted backwards nor forwards PFP1.	• Lubricant (water-soluble jelly or sterile water).	• Additional protective clothing may be necessary if indicated by the patient's condition (see Chapter 9).
	• pH strips.	
• Protect the patient's clothing with a towel.	• Receiver or vomit bowl.	
	• A 20/50 ml syringe PFP3.	
	• Two small gallipots.	
	• Adhesive tape, tissues, yellow waste bag.	

Procedure

1. Take the equipment to the bedside.

2. Agree with the patient a signal (e.g. hand signal) that can be used should he/she want the nurse to stop.

3. Estimate the length of tube to be inserted by measuring the distance from the patient's nose to the tip of the earlobe and then to the xiphisternum, and make a note of where this is on the tube (Figure 6.3) PFP4.

4. Ask/assist the patient to remove dentures and to clear nasal passages by blowing the nose. Select the best nostril (not tender, no deviated septum, etc.).

5. Encourage the patient to relax as much as possible and to breathe steadily.

6. Prepare the tube as per manufacturer's instructions (e.g. lubricating the tip of the tube and injecting sterile water down the tube to activate coating).

7. Pass the tube gently into the nostril and pass backwards (not upwards) along the floor of the nose to the nasopharynx. (If a blockage is felt, change to the other nostril.)

8. Pause to allow the patient to draw breath and recover.

9. Ask the patient to breathe through their mouth and swallow. As the patient swallows, and while keeping the head level, gently advance the tube. A sip of water may help the patient to 'swallow' the tube.

10. When the tube has reached the measured distance, check it is in the stomach by one or more of the following methods:
    • Aspirate a small amount of stomach contents (0.5–1 ml) from the tube. Apply aspirate to a pH strip, leave for 1 minute and then compare with the

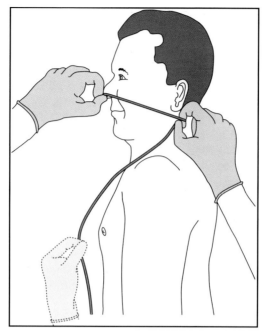

Figure 6.3 Measuring the length of tube to be inserted

colour bars to get a reading. A pH of 5.5 or less confirms gastric placement PFP5.

- If unable to obtain any aspirate or the pH is greater than 5.5, injecting 10–20 ml of air using a 20/50 ml syringe will dispel any residual fluid. Advance the tube by 10–20 cm, turn the patient onto their side, leave for 1 hour and try aspirating again. If the pH is still greater than 5.5 the position of the tube should be confirmed by X-ray. X-ray should be used to confirm the position of the tube in all unconscious patients PFP6.

11. Secure the tube ensuring that friction or pressure on the tip of the nose is avoided and the patient's vision is not obstructed.

Post procedure

Patient	Equipment/Environment	Nurse
• Ensure the patient is comfortable.	• Clear away the equipment. • Dispose of waste appropriately. • If a fine-bore tube has been used, remove the guide wire using gentle traction PFP7.	• Remove gloves and apron and wash hands. • Document nasogastric tube insertion and report any abnormal findings.

Points for practice

1. Insertion of the nasogastric tube may be for feeding or for gastric aspiration (Phillips 2006). The upright position is best for nasogastric tube insertion; if this is not possible, the patient should be lying on one side.

2. If the nasogastric tube is being inserted for the purpose of enteral feeding, a fine- or small-bore tube should be used. They reduce patient discomfort and provide a decreased risk of aspiration. They are also less likely to cause complications such as gastritis, oesophageal and nasal irritation. The wide bore (Ryles's tube) should only be used for gastric drainage, medication administration, gastric lavage and diagnostic testing (Phillips 2006).

3. Using a larger syringe allows gentle pressure and suction. A smaller syringe may produce too much pressure and split the tube. Polyurethane syringes are preferable to other syringes (National Patient Safety Agency 2005).

4. Having measured the tube, make a note of how much will remain outside the nose; the tube may have markings on it to facilitate this. It is important to measure the tube to ensure that it does not pass through the stomach and into the duodenum (Cannaby et al 2002).

5. A pH between 0 and 5.5 is seen as a safe cut-off when determining if the tube is in the stomach. According to the NSPA (2005) this range minimises the incidence of removing tubes that are actually in the stomach and reduces the undesirable increased use of X-ray.

6. Advancing the tube may allow it to pass from the oesophagus into the stomach. Flushing the tube with 10/20 ml of air will dispel any residual fluid (nasopharyngeal secretions/water) and may also dislodge the tip of the tube from the gastric mucosa. Turning the patient on their side will enable the tube to enter the gastric fluid pool. Changes to the pH strip may not occur in some clinical conditions (e.g. pernicious anaemia or previous gastrectomy) or if the patient is receiving H_2-receptor antagonists (which decrease the secretion of gastric acid) or if the tube has passed through the pylorus. X-ray should not be used routinely to check the position of the nasogastric tube. However, it is the method of choice in patients who are unconscious with no gag reflex. **The following methods must not be used to test the position of the tube**: auscultation, litmus paper tests, the 'whoosh test' (injecting air and listening for a bubbling sound) and absence of respiratory distress in the patient (NPSA 2005).

7. If an X-ray is required when a fine-bore tube has been inserted, the guide wire should not be removed until confirmation of its position in the stomach has been established. The guide wire is then removed by holding the tube at the nose with one hand and pulling the wire out with the other. If it is difficult to remove, then the tube should be removed as well. Do not reinsert the guide wire after removal, as there is a risk of perforation of the oesophageal or stomach wall.

NASOGASTRIC FEEDING

Preparation

Patient	Equipment/Environment	Nurse
• Explain the procedure, to gain consent and co-operation.	• Nasogastric feeding pump, or reservoir bottle or bag if a gravity method is being used.	• Wash and dry hands thoroughly.
• Ensure the patient is comfortable and sitting upright if condition permits.	• Prescribed nasogastric feed plus enteral administration set.	• Put on apron. Additional protective clothing may be necessary if indicated by the patient's condition (see Chapter 9).
	• 50 ml syringe and sterile water PFP1.	
	• 20 ml syringe, gallipot and pH strips to check tube position PFP2.	

Procedure

1. Take the equipment to the bedside.

2. Check the nasogastric tube is in the stomach, aspirating a small amount of stomach contents (0.5–1 ml) from the tube with a 20 ml syringe. Apply aspirate to a pH strip, leave for 1 minute and then compare to colour bars to get a reading. A pH of 5.5 or less confirms gastric placement (see page 120).

3. Flush the tube with 25–30 ml of water before commencing feed.

4. Remove the cap of the feed bottle and attach the administration set according to the manufacturer's instructions. If a separate reservoir is being used, pour the feed into the bag/reservoir and attach the administration set. (Sterile water may be given via this method.)

5. Allow the feed to run through the tubing to expel all air and then close the roller clamp.

6. Connect the administration set to the nasogastric tube securely.

7. If using a pump, insert the administration set according to the manufacturer's instructions and open the roller clamp. Switch the pump on (Figure 6.4), set it to the prescribed rate and press 'start'. If no pump is being used, adjust the roller clamp until the prescribed flow rate is achieved.

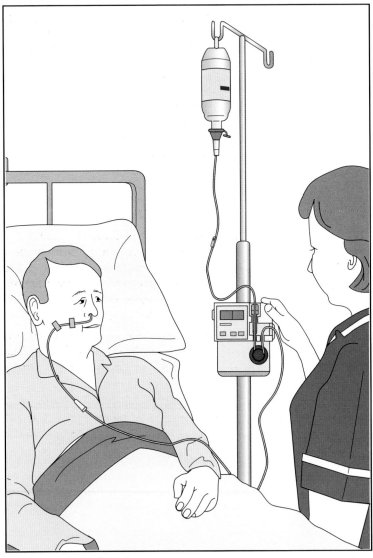

Figure 6.4 Nasogastric feeding via a pump

Post procedure

Patient	Equipment/Environment	Nurse
• Ensure the patient is comfortable and observe for signs of nausea, gastric reflux or dyspnoea. • Attend to the patient's hygiene (mouth, lips and nostrils) as necessary. • Observe for diarrhoea or constipation.	• Clear away the equipment and wipe up any spillages. • When the feed has finished, detach the bottle from the administration set and flush the nasogastric tube with at least 30 ml of sterile water to prevent stasis of feed in the tube **PFP3**. • Change the administration set every 24 hours. Attach label indicating date and time set up.	• Remove apron and wash hands. • Record the feed on the fluid balance chart and other relevant documentation. • Report any complications.

Points for practice

1. The size of syringe required to aspirate the tube will vary. If a fine-bore tube is used, a 20 ml syringe will be adequate. However, if a Ryles-type (large-bore) tube is used, it will not be possible to attach an ordinary syringe: a 50 ml catheter-tip syringe will be necessary. When aspirating, it is important to avoid creating too much suction, as being sucked against the end of the tube may damage the gastric mucosa (Cannaby et al 2002).

2. It is vital to check the position of the tube prior to each feed (see page 120). If a fine-bore tube is used, the patient may not always show signs of distress if the tube (and subsequently nasogastric feed) enters the lungs (Cannaby et al 2002).

3. If a second bottle of feed is due to commence, ensure that the first does not empty completely, allowing air to enter the administration set. If this does happen, the set will need to be disconnected and primed again before the second feed can commence.

CARE OF GASTROSTOMY SITE

Principles

- There are different types of gastrostomy tubes, some of which lie flush with the skin and others that protrude. There are those that have a one-way valve to prevent reflux and a silicone dome that acts as an internal anchoring device. Others have an external skin disc and an internal balloon that anchors the device (Holmes 2004).

- The tube should be secure but not too tight. If the internal or external part of the tube is too tight against the abdominal wall it can cause severe discomfort and cellulitis and bleeding (Green and Jackson 2006).

- The main disadvantage of percutaneous endoscopic gastrostomy (PEG) is the risk of wound infection due to contamination by oral flora during insertion. Therefore, the site should be treated as a wound after insertion and prophylactic antibiotics are usually prescribed (Holmes 2004).

- Care of the wound site involves ensuring it remains clean and dry. Serosanguinous drainage can be expected in the first 7–10 days (Holmes 2004). Although local practices may vary, most policies recommend that the site is cleaned with sterile 0.9% sodium chloride, although sterile water is also adequate. The site can be sprayed with an iodine-based powder spray, and a sterile, occlusive and moisture permeable dressing applied.

- The dressing should be changed twice weekly unless the stoma is discharging, in which case it should be changed daily. If gastric juices leak through the dressing they can cause irritation. To protect the skin from excoriation, a skin barrier wafer sealed at the inner edge with karaya gum can be used (Holmes 2004). When the area has healed, no dressing is necessary.

- The site should be observed for signs of inflammation, excoriation and gastric leakage, and the patient's temperature and pulse rate should be monitored for 7 days. If infection at the insertion site becomes evident, careful cleansing with soap and water or antibacterial solutions and the application of a topical antibiotic is necessary (NICE 2006).

- Once the site has healed, the guard surrounding the tube (Figure 6.5) should be lifted up daily and slid round the tube so that the area can be washed with warm soapy water and then dried thoroughly. The tube should then be rotated, to prevent necrosis caused by pressure from the balloon inside the stomach. The guard is then replaced.

- It is recommended that the patient shower rather than bathe, as the stoma site should not be immersed in water until it is healed (Howell 2002). The gastrostomy tube should be closed while the patient is showering or bathing and the site dried thoroughly afterwards.

- Feeding can be commenced 4 hours after insertion when it is safe and well tolerated (Howell 2002), although this may be longer if the patient has had a

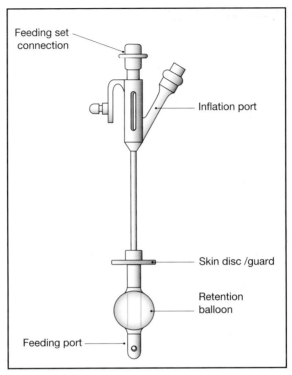

Feeding set connection

Inflation port

Skin disc /guard

Retention balloon

Feeding port

Figure 6.5 A gastrostomy tube

general anaesthetic as gastric function may be disrupted. The presence or absence of bowel sounds to initiate feeding is debated. Although bowel sounds should be present, Loan et al (1998) state that bowel sounds indicate gastric motility, not absorption and suggest that feeding should not be dependent on bowel sounds. Abdominal distension and pain are more pertinent indicators of whether to withhold feeds.

- The most common cause of blockage of the tube is inadequate flushing. The tube should be flushed with 25–30 ml of sterile water at least twice daily if the feeds are continuous, before and after feeds and the administration of drugs. Tubes placed in the jejunum require 4 hourly flushing (British Association for Parenteral and Enteral Nutrition (BAPEN) 2003).

FEEDING VIA PERCUTANEOUS ENDOSCOPIC GASTROSTOMY (PEG)

Preparation

Patient	Equipment/Environment	Nurse
• Explain the procedure, to gain consent and co-operation PFP1.	• Prescription chart and prescribed feed.	• Wash and dry hands thoroughly.
• It is advisable for the patient to be sitting up (unless the feed is given very slowly) PFP2.	• Enteral feed administration set.	• Put on apron. Additional protective clothing may be necessary if indicated by the patient's condition (see Chapter 9).
• Bowel sounds should be present PFP3.	• Syringe and 20–30 ml of sterile water (to flush tube).	
	• Enteral feed pump.	
	• Infusion stand.	
	• Fluid balance chart.	

Procedure

1. Take the equipment and the feed to the bedside and check the patient's name band.

2. Remove the cap of the feed bottle.

3. Maintaining asepsis, open the enteral feed administration set, attach it to the bottle according to the manufacturer's instructions, and close the flow control roller clamp PFP4.

4. Attach the hanger to the feed container and hang the feed container on the infusion stand.

5. Open the roller clamp on the administration set, allow the feed to run through to expel all air and then close the clamp. The plastic cap on the end of the administration set should remain in place so that the tube remains sterile.

6. Draw up 25–30 ml (depending on local policy) of sterile water and flush the tube PFP5.

7. Insert the administration set into the pump according to the manufacturer's instructions, remove the plastic cap at the distal end of it and attach it to the PEG tube.

8. Open the roller clamp and turn on the pump.

9. Set the flow rate as prescribed (e.g. 125 ml per hour) and start the pump.

10. Check that the feed is running, it is not leaking at the connection with the PEG tube, and that the tube is not kinked or blocked.

Post procedure

Patient	Equipment/Environment	Nurse
• Ensure the patient is comfortable. Observe PEG site regularly PFP6. • Return regularly, to check the feed is running satisfactorily. • Observe the patient for nausea, vomiting or diarrhoea.	• Clear away equipment and wipe up any spillages, especially on the pump. • On completion of the feed, disconnect the administration set and flush the tube with sterile water according to local policy PFP7. • The pump usually has alarms to indicate when the feed has finished or if the tube has become blocked or kinked. • If there are no alarms, extra checking is required.	• Remove apron and wash hands. • Document the type of feed, time started, rate of flow and volume of water used to flush the tube.

Points for practice

1. As eating and drinking are social activities as well as physical necessities, it is important to try and make PEG/gastrostomy feeds as pleasant and 'normal' as possible, e.g. if the feed is not continuous, by administering the feed when others are eating their meals.

2. Feeding via a PEG tube may be intermittent or continuous. Continuous feeding has been shown to reduce the incidence of diarrhoea (Howell 2002).

3. Bowel sounds should be present before feeding via the PEG is commenced, although the decision to commence feeding should not be based entirely on their presence (Loan et al 1998) (see page 127).

4. Avoid adding anything to the feed. If drugs are to be administered via the PEG tube, they must be soluble in water and the tube should be flushed with 25–30 ml of sterile water before and after their administration to prevent blockage (BAPEN 2003).

5. When flushing the PEG tube, care should be taken when attaching the syringe, to avoid damaging the connection. A 20 ml (or larger) syringe should be used to flush the tube, as the pressure exerted by smaller syringes is too great. If the PEG tube is not being used for feeding for a period of time, it should be flushed twice a day to maintain patency (Holmes 2004).

6. The site should be inspected daily for signs of leakage, swelling, skin irritation or breakdown, soreness or excessive movement of the tube.

7. The administration set must be changed every 24 hours and should be labelled to indicate the date that the change is due.

References and further reading

Anderson B. (2005) Nutrition and wound healing: the necessity of assessment. *British Journal of Nursing (Tissue Viability Supplement)* **14**(19):S30–S38.

This article explores protein depletion as a result of malnutrition and considers its importance in respect of wound healing.

Barton A, Fuller R, Dudley N. (2004) Using subcutaneous fluids to rehydrate older people: current practice and future challenges. *Oxford Journal of Medicine* **97**:765–768.

This article is a review of the evidence for the use of subcutaneous fluids in the hospital setting. Future possible development in respect of drug administration and the use of subcutaneous fluids for older people in long-term residential settings are considered.

Brogden B. (2004) Clinical skills: importance of nutrition for acutely ill hospital patients. *British Journal of Nursing* **13**(15):914–920.

This article provides an overview of the metabolic changes that occur during starvation in health and illness and a review of a range of nutrition support options is presented and indications for their use provided.

Cannaby AM, Evans L, Freeman A. (2002) Nursing care of patients with nasogastric feeding tubes. *British Journal of Nursing* **11**(6):366–372.

This article focuses on a small scale study and indicates differences in the care of patients with nasogastric feeding tubes. The article provides a useful overview of recommended practice.

Department of Health. (2003) *The essence of care.* DoH, London.

The Essence of Care launched in February 2001 provides a tool to help practitioners take a patient-focused and structured approach to sharing and comparing practice. It enabled healthcare personnel to work with patients to identify best practice and to develop action plans to improve care. Food and nutrition is one of the eight benchmarks of care.

Grieve RJ, Finnie A. (2002) Nutritional care: implications and recommendations for nursing. *British Journal of Nursing* **11**(7):432–437.

This article explores why current nutritional care in nursing practice is often inadequate. It offers implications of such practice and proposes recommendations for future change.

Holmes S. (2003) Undernutrition in hospital patients. *Nursing Standard* **17**(19):45–52.

This article is part of the Continuing Professional Development Series and gives a comprehensive overview of the issues related to under-nutrition in hospital and its impact on patients. The article also focuses on the role of nutrition in good clinical practice.

Holmes S. (2004) Enteral feeding and percutaneous endoscopic gastrostomy. *Nursing Standard* **18**(20):41–43.

This article reviews enteral feeding focusing on PEG and considers the after care and complications of this method of feeding.

Holmes S. (2006) Barriers to effective nutritional care for older adults. *Nursing Standard* **21**(3):50–54.

Although this article focuses on the older person, the issues identified are pertinent for the majority of hospitalised patients. The barriers to achieving nutritional adequacy once patients have been admitted to hospital are considered and suggestions for overcoming them are made.

Howell M. (2002) Do nurses know enough about percutaneous endoscopic gastrostomy? *Nursing Times* **98**(17):40–42.

This article reports on the results of an audit of PEG management. This article is useful as it incorporates recommended practice throughout.

Loan T, Magnuson B, Williams S. (1998) Debunking six myths about enteral feeding. *Nursing* **28**(8):43–48.

Although this article is older, it provides a very useful discussion of practices that are common but for which there is little evidence.

Mansfield S. (1998) Subcutaneous fluid administration and site maintenance. *Nursing Standard* **13**(12):56,59,60,62.

This article explores the practice associated with the use of hypodermoclysis as a means of fluid administration for older people in one Trust. Current practice was audited and practice guidelines formulated.

Moriarty D, Hudson E. (2001) Hypodermoclysis for rehydration in the community. *British Journal of Community Nursing* **6**(9):437–443.

Although the article focuses on the process of developing practice guidelines for community staff caring for patients receiving subcutaneous fluids for rehydration, it includes the background to the use of hypodermoclysis, its advantages, its indications for use with older people and those receiving palliative care as well as addressing some of the potential ethical issues.

National Institute for Health and Clinical Excellence. (2002) *Nutrition Support in Adults (Clinical Guideline 32)*. NICE, London.

This guideline is essential reading as it addresses all aspects of nutritional support using the best available evidence (www.nice.org.uk).

Phillips NM. (2006) Nasogastric tubes: an historical context. *Medsurg Nursing* **15**(2):84–88.

Although presented in a historical context this article does provide some useful insight into current practice.

Ross JR, Saunders Y, Cochrane M, Zepetella G. (2002) A prospective, within-patient comparison between metal butterfly needles and Teflon cannulae in subcutaneous infusion of drugs to terminally ill hospice patients. *Palliative Medicine* **16**:13–16.

This article outlines the results of a study undertaken to compare metal butterfly needles and Teflon cannulae.

Royal College of Nursing. (2003) *Standards for infusion therapy*. RCN, London.

This document provides a comprehensive overview and best practice guidance on all aspects of intravenous and subcutaneous infusion therapy including: infection control and safety, equipment, site selection, site care and complications.

Websites

British Association for Parenteral and Enteral Nutrition. (2003) *Administering drugs via enteral feeding tubes*. www.bapen.org.uk

This is a useful website for exploring multiple aspects of parenteral and enteral nutrition.

National Patient Safety Agency. (2005) *Reducing the harm caused by misplaced nasogastric feeding tubes*. www.npsa.nhs.uk/advice

This site is useful for keeping updated on many safety issues. In this instance there are clear guidelines about assessing the position of the nasogastric tube.

Notes

7

Medicines

STORAGE OF MEDICINES

Principles

In line with legal requirements and local policies, it is part of the nurse's role to ensure that medicines are safely stored. The following principles apply to all situations involving the storage and administration of medicines:

- All medicines, lotions and reagents (except intravenous fluids and drugs for use in emergency situations) must be stored in locked cupboards. Drugs for emergency use (e.g. in cardiac arrest) may be kept with the emergency equipment, but must be in a sealed container, which is then replenished and resealed after use.

- All medicines, including emergency drugs and intravenous fluids, must be stored in an environment that meets the manufacturers' recommendations, e.g. minimum or maximum temperature.

- Medicine cupboards must be kept locked at all times; drug trolleys must be locked and secured to the wall when not in use, and individual medicines cabinets (sometimes called 'patient's own dispensary') must be locked when not in use.

- Controlled drugs must be kept separate from other medicines, and the keys to the controlled drugs cupboard kept separately from other drug keys. A controlled drugs register must also be kept.

- All stock must be rotated so that medicines are used before their expiry date. Regular checks of stored medication must be made to ensure that stock rotation is effective.

- The security of medicines is the responsibility of the nurse in charge of the clinical area. No unauthorised person must be allowed access to the keys (refer to local policy regarding who has authorised access to the keys).

SELF-ADMINISTRATION

Principles

In some hospitals and care homes patients/residents (hereafter called patients) are given responsibility for taking their own prescribed medicines. This may be in preparation for their discharge home or to maintain their independence. Local policies will differ, but the principles for self-administration of medicines are based upon the availability of suitable storage (usually locked cupboards attached to the patient's locker or in their room), a medicines regimen that is not subject to frequent change and individually dispensed medicines from the pharmacy. The medicines may be dispensed in separate packs or in compliance aids such as a monitored dose container or a daily/weekly dosing aid:

- The nurse's role in self-administration of medicines is to support and educate the patient in the safe administration of their medicines and in the use of any compliance aids that may be used. In some instances it may be the nurse's role to support and educate carers or support workers in this role rather than the patient themselves.

- Collaborative working between all members of the healthcare team is imperative if the individual's suitability for self-administration is to be assessed and appropriate education and support provided.

- The nurse must assess the patient's ability to self-administer their medicines prior to entering them into the programme. Most policies for self-administration of medicines include obtaining written consent from the patient before entering them into the programme.

- Many programmes also have varying levels of supervision according to the patient's ability and the level of support and education required. For example, initially the nurse may administer the patient's medicines whilst implementing a planned programme of education. The education programme should include detailed information (both verbal and written) about the medicines, their dosage and times for administration, intended effects and any possible side effects. The written information should include patient information leaflets and also an individualised card indicating the times and dosages for each medicine. During this period the nurse can assess the need for any compliance aids that may be required, such as bottle-top openers or large print on labels. The next level of supervision is when patients administer their own medicines under supervision. The final level is when patients administer their own medicines and are given responsibility for the key to their cabinet. It is important that sufficient time is allocated to the programme, so that patients have time to fully understand their medicines prior to discharge home or the implementation of the programme in a residential home.

- It is important to reassess the patient's ability to self-administer medications at frequent intervals.
- Nurses may find that, in some instances, they have to take responsibility for repackaging dispensed medicines into compliance aids for patients. This must be undertaken with care and the nurse must be aware of the risk of error in this procedure (NMC 2006). The procedure must be documented and all medicines must be accounted for.

DRUG CALCULATIONS

It is sometimes necessary to carry out drug calculations in order to administer prescribed medicines correctly, for example, when the medicines are not available in the exact dosage that has been prescribed.

Converting from one unit of measurement to another

It is sometimes necessary to convert from one unit of measurement to another in order to be able to administer the correct amount of medicine.

To convert units you need to know the following:

$$1 \text{ kilogram (kg)} = 1000 \text{ grams (g)}$$
$$1 \text{ gram (g)} = 1000 \text{ milligrams (mg)}$$
$$1 \text{ milligram} = 1000 \text{ micrograms (mcg)}$$

To convert grams (g) to milligrams (mg) or milligrams (mg) to micrograms (mcg) you need to multiply by 1000. This is achieved by moving the decimal point three places to the right, e.g.:

$$6.5\text{mg} \times 1000 = 6500\text{mcg}$$

To convert micrograms (mcg) into milligrams (mg) or milligrams (mg) to grams (g), you need to divide by 1000. This is achieved by moving the decimal point three places to the left, e.g.:

$$2500\text{mcg} = 2.5\text{mg}$$

Percentage concentration and ratios

Sometimes drug concentration may be measured as a percentage (%) weight to volume (w/v). The percentage equates to the number of grams (weight) per 100 millilitres (volume), i.e.:

1% lignocaine equates to 1g of lignocaine dissolved in every 100ml
5% glucose equates to 5g of glucose dissolved in every 100ml

The percentage remains constant irrespective of the size of the container.

Occasionally drug concentrations are written as ratios. The ratio 1:1000 equates to 1g per 1000ml and the ratio: 1:10,000 equates to 1g per 10,000ml.

e.g. adrenaline (epinephrine) 1:1000 (1g per 1000ml)
$$= 1000\text{mg per } 1000\text{ml}$$
$$= 1\text{mg per ml}$$

e.g. adrenaline (epinephrine) 1:10,000 (1g per 10,000ml)
$$= 1000\text{mg per} 10,000\text{ml}$$
$$= 1\text{mg per } 10\text{ml}$$
$$= 0.1\text{mg per ml}$$

Calculating the number of tablets required

In order to calculate the correct number of tablets, use the following formula:

$$\text{number of measures required (i.e. tablets)} = \frac{\text{dose prescribed}}{\text{dose per measure}}$$

Firstly you need to convert the amount required into the same units of measurement as the tablets, then use the formula.

For example, 1 g of paracetamol is prescribed. Paracetamol is dispensed in 500 mg tablets:

$$1g = 1000mg$$

$$\text{Number of tablets} = \frac{1000mg}{500mg}$$

$$= 2 \text{ tablets to be given}$$

Calculating the volume to give

In order to calculate the correct volume, use the following formula:

$$\text{volume to give} = \frac{\text{dose required}}{\text{dose available}} \times \text{volume available}$$

For example, 75mg of pethidine is prescribed. Pethidine is dispensed in ampoules containing 100mg in 2ml:

$$\text{volume to give} = \frac{75}{100} \times 2 = 1.5ml$$

Calculating infusion rates

See 'Intravenous therapy', 'Regulation of flow rate' (page 78).

PRINCIPLES OF ADMINISTRATION

The following principles apply to the administration of all medicines, regardless of route.

Preparation

Patient

- Check the location of the patient before dispensing the medication. Do not leave medicines unattended for administration at a later time.
- Check the patient understands the reasons for the medication being administered and any special instructions, e.g. swallow whole or after food, etc. Ensure that they consented to receiving the medicine **PFP1**.
- Ascertain whether the patient has any drug allergies **PFP2**.
- The patient should be wearing an identification wrist band.

Equipment/Environment

- Medicines to be administered and equipment appropriate to the route of administration.
- Patient's prescription chart.
- Drug reference book, e.g. British National Formulary.

Nurse

- **Medicines may only be administered by a registered nurse PFP3.**
- The nurse must have knowledge of the action, usual dose and side effects of the drugs being administered and knowledge of legislation and local policies relating to the administration of medicines (NMC 2004).
- Local policy may require that two nurses check certain medicines before administration.
- Wash and dry hands thoroughly.

Procedure

1. Check the prescription chart has patient's full name and hospital number and read the prescription to ascertain which medicines require administration **PFP4**.
2. Check by which route each medicine is to be given.
3. Check the prescription is dated and is legible and signed by an authorised prescriber **PFP5**.
4. Check it is the correct time to administer the medicine and that the patient has not already received it. Check any special observations (e.g. blood pressure or pulse rate) or requirements relating to the medication (e.g. before or after food).
5. Identify the correct medication by checking the medicine container against the prescription chart.

6. Check the expiry date of the medicine.

7. Calculate how much is needed to achieve the prescribed dose (e.g. how many tablets or how much of the ampoule is to be drawn up) **PFP6**.

8. Repeat steps 2–7 for all medicines due at this time.

9. Check the patient's identity – using the patient's nameband, a photograph or verbally, against the prescription chart, according to local policy **PFP7**.

10. Administer the medicine as prescribed. **Medicines must not be left at the bedside unattended**. The patient may forget to take them or another patient may take them by mistake.

Post procedure

Patient	Equipment/Environment	Nurse
• Ensure the patient is comfortable and understands why the medication has been administered.	• Dispose of any packaging and other waste.	• Sign/initial the prescription chart according to local policy, to indicate that the medicine has been administered. If the medication cannot be administered for some reason, this must also be documented.
		• Monitor the effects of the medication and document in the nursing records. Report any abnormal effects/side effects immediately.

Points for practice

1. Except in exceptional circumstances, medicines for patients who refuse to take them should not be given covertly by disguising them in food (NMC 2006).

2. If the allergy section of the prescription chart has not been completed, check with the patient and/or the medical notes before administering any medicines. If the patient has no known allergies, this should be indicated in the box, it should not just be left blank.

3. Student nurses may only participate in the administration of medicines under the direct supervision of a registered nurse. A registered nurse must countersign all student signatures.

4. Patient Group Directions (PGDs) are sometimes used in lieu of an individual prescription. These are written instructions for the supply or administration of

medicines to groups of patients. They must be signed by a doctor or dentist AND a pharmacist who have been involved in developing them AND they must be approved by the appropriate healthcare body, e.g. an Acute Healthcare Trust or Primary Care Trust. Some employers require specific training for those who use PGDs and so local policy must be followed (NMC 2006).

5. Instruction by telephone to administer a previously unprescribed substance is not acceptable. In exceptional circumstances, where the authorised prescriber is unable to issue a new prescription for an altered dose of an existing prescription, fax or e-mail may be used. This must be followed up with a new prescription confirming the new prescription. The Nursing and Midwifery Council (2006) suggest that this should be within 24 hours.

6. If the dosage of medication is related to weight, the patient's weight should be recorded on the prescription chart.

7. To reduce the risk of error all patients should wear an identification wrist band. If checking their identity verbally it is important to ask them to state their name and date of birth.

ORAL ROUTE

Preparation

Patient	Equipment/Environment	Nurse
• Ask/assist the patient to assume a position that allows easy swallowing.	• Medicines to be administered plus medicine pots, tablet cutter, tissues, jug of water and/or milk if appropriate.	• **Only registered nurses may administer medicines** `PFP1`.
• Ensure the patient has plenty of appropriate fluid with which to take the medicine.	• Prescription chart.	• Wash and dry hands thoroughly.
		• Additional protective clothing may be necessary if indicated by the patient's condition (see Chapter 9).

Procedure

1. Check the prescription as described on page 139.

2. Calculate how much liquid or how many tablets or capsules are required to achieve the prescribed dose (see page 138). Do not break tablets unless they are scored across the middle. Break scored tablets with a file, tablet cutter or using a tissue, to avoid handling `PFP2`.

3. Dispense the prescribed amount into a medicine pot. If not in a blister pack, shake the tablets/capsules into the top of the container before transferring to the medicine pot, to avoid handling them (Figure 7.1). Liquid preparations may be drawn up in a syringe for accuracy of measurement and then transferred into a medicines pot or the liquid can be squirted from the syringe directly into the patient's mouth.

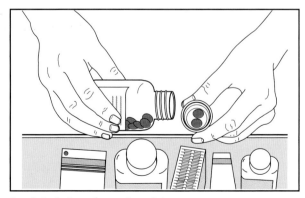

Figure 7.1 Non-touch technique for oral medicines

4. Repeat this procedure for all medicines due at this time.

5. Check the patient's identity – using the patient's nameband or verbally, according to local policy – against the prescription chart.

6. Make sure the patient is in an appropriate position to swallow the medicine and has sufficient fluid.

7. Watch or assist the patient to take the medicines. **Do not leave medicines unattended at the bedside** for later administration.

Post procedure

Patient	Equipment/Environment	Nurse
• Make sure the patient has taken the medicine as prescribed **PFP3**.	• Dispose of any packaging, disposable medicine pots, etc., in the clinical waste. • Wash and dry other equipment as necessary and leave ready for use.	• Document drugs administered according to local policy.

Points for practice

1. Student nurses may only participate in the administration of medicines under the direct supervision of a registered nurse. A registered nurse must countersign all student signatures.

2. Only soluble or dispersible preparations may be dissolved in water. If the patient is unable to swallow whole tablets, the pharmacist should be consulted to identify an alternative preparation, e.g. suspension or elixir. Tablets should not be crushed as this may alter the chemical properties of the medication. Additionally, crushing a tablet usually renders it 'unlicensed' and as such the manufacturer will not assume any liability (NMC 2006). Medication must only be crushed with the permission of the authorised prescriber and pharmacist and with the patient's consent. The reasons for crushing the medication must also be clearly documented.

3. Except in exceptional circumstances, medicines for patients who refuse to take them should not be given covertly by disguising them in food (NMC 2006).

NASOGASTRIC ROUTE

Some patients are unable to take nourishment and medicines orally. If they have a nasogastric tube, medicines may be administered via this route. It is imperative that the pharmacist is consulted to determine whether tablets may be crushed and mixed with water or whether alternative solutions, such as suspensions and elixirs, are available (see page 143 regarding crushing tablets). You should also consider whether any interaction with the feed may occur and the possibility of blockage of the tube (Best 2005). See nasogastric feeding (page 123) for technique.

CONTROLLED DRUGS

Preparation

Patient	Equipment/Environment	Nurse
• Explain the procedure, to gain consent and co-operation.	• Patient's prescription chart.	• Ensure knowledge of legislation and local policies relating to the administration of controlled drugs PFP1 & 2.
• Check the patient understands the reasons for having the medication.	• Controlled drugs register.	• Two nurses are usually required, one of whom must be a registered nurse (check local policy).
		• Wash and dry hands thoroughly.
		• Additional protective clothing may be necessary if indicated by the patient's condition (see Chapter 9).

Procedure

If local policy stipulates two nurses, they must both be involved in all stages of this procedure:

1. Read the prescription chart to ascertain which drugs require administration and by which route.

2. Check that the prescription has the patient's full name and hospital number and is dated, legible and signed by the authorised prescriber.

3. Check that it is the correct time to administer the drug and that the patient has not already received it. You may also need to check that the appropriate time has elapsed since the previous dose and any special requirements, such as the maximum dosage allowed in 24 hours.

4. Select the appropriate drug from the controlled drugs cupboard, checking that the quantity corresponds with that indicated in the controlled drugs register. Check the expiry date.

5. Remove the drug from its container and check it against the prescription.

6. Check the quantity remaining and replace in the cupboard. Lock the cupboard.

7. Check the amount required, route, time and patient's identity again with the prescription.

8. Select/draw up the correct amount/volume of the drug, performing any calculation as required. Any unused drug should be discarded into a sharps bin PFP3.

9. In the controlled drugs register, record the patient's full name, the dose to be administered (any wastage must also be recorded), the time and the stock number remaining.

10. At the bedside, check that the information on the patient's nameband corresponds with that on the prescription. Check again the drug, dose, route and time against the prescription.

11. Administer the drug by the prescribed route. Both nurses must now sign the prescription chart and the controlled drugs register.

Post procedure

Patient

- Ensure the patient is comfortable and is aware of the effects and side effects of the drug.

Equipment/Environment

- Discard all waste appropriately.
- Ensure the controlled drugs register is completed and returned to the appropriate place **PFP4**.

Nurse

- Monitor the effects of the drug and report any side effects immediately.

Points for practice

1. The keys to the controlled drugs cupboard must be kept separately from other keys and must be carried by the registered nurse in charge of the ward. No unauthorised personnel must have access to these keys.

2. Some drugs are controlled drugs in certain preparations only. For example, intramuscular dihydrocodeine (DF118) is a controlled drug but the oral preparation is not.

3. It is important to ensure that any unused drug is discarded safely and cannot be used by unauthorised persons. Previous advice was to wash it down the sink, but it is now recommended that it should be discarded into a sharps bin as even small traces of drugs can have an adverse effect on the environment.

4. Controlled-drug registers must not be thrown away when full, but must be retained in storage for 5 years. Check local policy for details.

SUBCUTANEOUS INJECTION

Preparation

Patient	Equipment/Environment	Nurse
• Explain the procedure, to gain consent and co-operation. • Ask/assist the patient to choose the site of injection.	• Prescription chart. • Prescribed drug (this is often a pre-filled syringe with needle). • Cardboard tray or receiver. • Syringe of appropriate size (0.5–2 ml) if necessary **PFP1**. • Orange (25G) needle if necessary. • Small clinical wipe/tissue. • Sharps bin.	• **Only registered nurses may administer medicines** **PFP2**. • Knowledge of local drug administration policy. • Wash and dry hands thoroughly. • Protective clothing may be necessary if indicated by the patient's condition (see Chapter 9).

Procedure

1. Check the drug against the prescription (see page 139) and check the patient's nameband.

2. If it is not a pre-filled syringe, prepare the medication as for intramuscular injection (see page 150) **PFP3**.

3. Select the site of administration (Figure 7.2) **PFP4**.

4. It is not necessary to clean the skin **PFP5**. Pinch up the skin using the thumb and first finger of your non-dominant hand and insert the short needle into the subcutaneous tissue at an angle of 80–90° (Figure 7.3A) **PFP6**.

5. It is not necessary to withdraw the piston as it is unlikely that a blood vessel of any size will be punctured.

6. Inject the solution slowly. On completion, pause briefly before withdrawing the needle as this helps to prevent backtracking.

7. Do not massage the site **PFP7**. If necessary, use the tissue to wipe away any blood.

8. Dispose of the syringe and needle into the sharps bin immediately (see page 249). **Do not re-sheathe the needle.**

Post procedure

Patient	Equipment/Environment	Nurse
• Ensure the patient is comfortable and is aware of the effects and side effects of the drug.	• Put away all equipment. Some drugs (e.g. insulin) have to be kept in the refrigerator. • Dispose of waste appropriately.	• Sign the prescription to indicate that the drug has been administered. • Report any abnormalities/ complications.

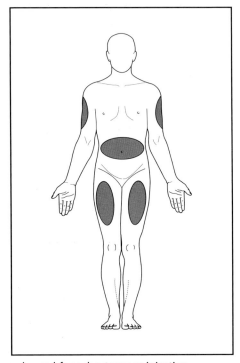

Figure 7.2 Sites commonly used for subcutaneous injection

Points for practice

1. No more that 2 ml should be given by the subcutaneous route.

2. **Only registered nurses may administer medications**. Student nurses may only participate in the administration of medicines under the direct supervision of a registered nurse. A registered nurse must countersign student signatures.

3. Some drugs (e.g. heparin) are manufactured in pre-filled syringes. Unlike all other injections, the air in a heparin syringe is not expelled, but is designed to remain in the syringe, next to the piston. When the small amount of drug is given, the air fills the needle hub/nozzle of the syringe and needle ensuring that all fluid has been expelled from the syringe. This prevents the drug tracking back to the surface as the needle is withdrawn, which can cause skin irritation.

4. Patients receiving regular subcutaneous injections (e.g. insulin) should rotate the injection site; repeated injections into the same area causes hardening of the subcutaneous tissues, which will interfere with absorption (King 2003). Possible sites are: the upper arms, the anterior aspect of the thighs, and the abdomen (see Figure 7.2). Heparin is usually given into the subcutaneous tissue of the abdominal wall.

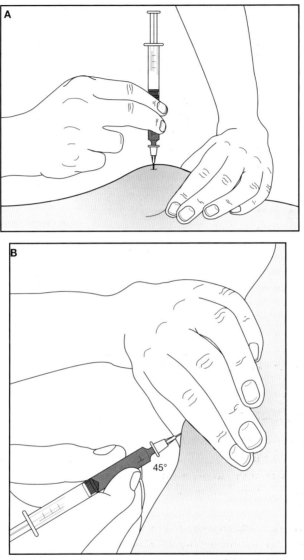

Figure 7.3 (A) Subcutaneous injection technique at 90° angle; (B) subcutaneous injection technique at 45° angle.

5. The skin is not cleaned because, with repeated use, alcohol causes the skin to harden and many patients will be having subcutaneous injections over a long period of time, possibly for the rest of their life.

6. If not using a pre-filled syringe or insulin 'pen', the needle will be longer than 5–8 mm; longer needles should be inserted at an angle of 45° (see Figure 7.3B).

7. Massaging the skin affects the absorption of the drug (Court & Lamb 1997).

INTRAMUSCULAR INJECTION

Preparation

Patient	Equipment/Environment	Nurse
• Explain the procedure, to gain consent and co-operation.	• Prescription chart.	• Only registered nurses may administer medicines. A second nurse may be required depending on the local drug administration policy PFP2.
• Check the patient's understanding of the reason for the injection.	• Prescribed medicine and diluent if required.	
	• Cardboard tray or receiver.	
	• Sterile syringe of appropriate size (2–5 ml).	
	• Sterile needle – usually green (21G) for adult patients PFP1.	• Wash and dry hands thoroughly.
	• Alcohol-impregnated swab.	• Gloves may be required depending on the type of drug being given (e.g. antibiotics).
	• Small clinical wipe/tissue.	
	• Sharps bin.	

Procedure

1. Check the medicine and any diluent against the prescription chart and check expiry dates (see checking procedure, page 139).

2. Open the syringe packaging at the plunger end and remove the syringe. Check that the plunger will move freely inside the barrel.

3. Taking care not to touch the nozzle end, hold the syringe in one hand and open the needle packaging at the hilt (coloured) end. Attach the needle firmly to the syringe and loosen, but do not remove, the needle cover (sheath). Place in the tray/receiver.

4. If a glass ampoule of liquid is being used, ensure that all the contents are in the bottom of the ampoule, then break off the top using a clinical wipe/tissue or syringe wrapper to protect your fingers. If a plastic ampoule is being used, break off the top, taking care not to touch the top of the ampoule with your fingers.

5. Pick up the syringe and needle and allow the needle cover to slide off into the tray or receiver.

6. Carefully insert the needle through the neck of the ampoule and into the solution, taking care not to allow it to scrape against the bottom of the ampoule, as this blunts the needle.

7. Draw back on the plunger, using your thumb and middle finger on the plunger with your first finger against the flange of the syringe until the required amount is in the syringe (see Figure 7.4).

8. If the medicine is in powder form, draw up the diluent, clean the rubber stopper of the ampoule/vial with an alcohol-impregnated swab and allow it to

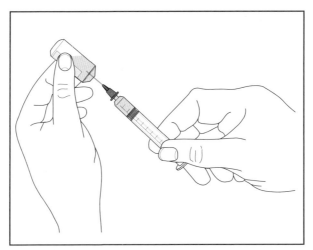

Figure 7.4 Drawing up the injection

dry. Inject the appropriate amount of diluent (see manufacturer's instructions; usually 1.5–2 ml) into the ampoule/vial. Mix thoroughly by gently agitating or rolling the ampoule/vial until all the powder has dissolved **PFP3**.

9. Holding the ampoule/vial upside down at eye level, pull back the plunger to draw the liquid into the syringe. Make sure that the needle remains below the surface of the liquid to prevent air being drawn into the syringe (**Figure** 7.4).

10. Replace the ampoule in tray/receiver. Taking care not to touch the needle with your hand, carefully resheathe the needle using the non-touch method (**Figure** 7.5) **PFP4**.

11. Hold the syringe upright at eye level and encourage any air to rise to the top of the syringe. Gently tap the barrel of the syringe if necessary to make air bubbles rise to the top. Expel the air by gently pressing the plunger until droplets of liquid are seen at the top of the needle (**Figure** 7.6).

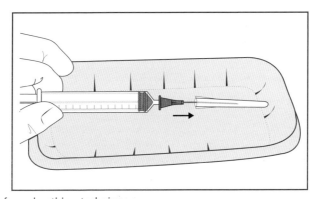

Figure 7.5 Safe re-sheathing technique

12. Take the tray/receiver containing the syringe, ampoule and alcohol-impregnated swab plus the sharps bin to the patient. Check the medicine and prescription again and the patient's nameband.

13. Ensure privacy. Select the site and ask/assist the patient to adopt a suitable position (Figure 7.7) **PFP5**.

14. Clean the skin with the alcohol-impregnated swab and allow it to dry **PFP6**.

15. Stretch the skin slightly with your non-dominant hand.

16. Holding the syringe like a dart in your dominant hand, warn the patient, then insert the needle swiftly and firmly at an angle of 90° to the skin (see Figure 7.8). Leave 0.5–1 cm of the needle showing **PFP7**.

17. With the ulnar border of your hand against the skin, hold the coloured part of the needle to prevent movement.

18. Withdraw the plunger slightly to check the needle has not inadvertently entered a blood vessel **PFP8**.

19. Depress the plunger steadily, not too quickly, until the syringe is empty.

20. Quickly and smoothly withdraw the needle from the skin and press firmly on the site with the swab or a tissue until any bleeding stops.

21. **Do not resheathe the needle.** Discard it, still attached to the syringe, into the sharps bin **PFP9**.

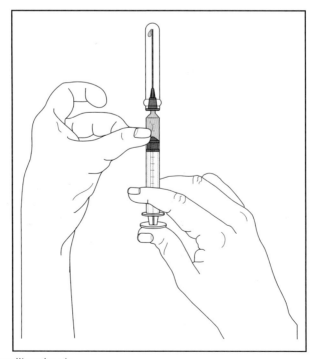

Figure 7.6 Expelling the air

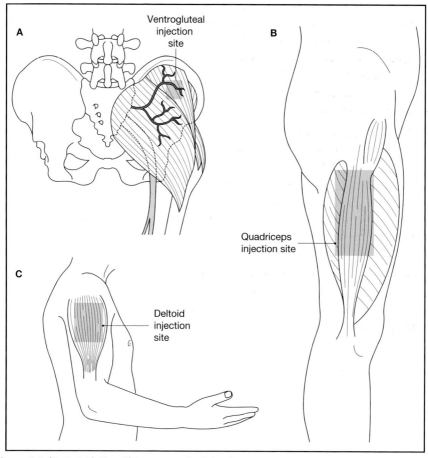

Figure 7.7 (A, B & C) Sites if intramuscular injection

Post procedure

Patient

- Assist the patient into a comfortable position and replace clothing as necessary.
- Intramuscular medicines given will usually take effect within 20 minutes. Check for the desired effect and for side effects, especially if an analgesic or anti-emetic.

Equipment/Environment

- Discard all used equipment appropriately.

Nurse

- Wash hands.
- Sign/initial the prescription chart to indicate that the medicine has been given.

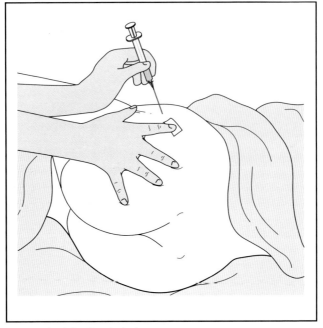

Figure 7.8 Intramuscular injection technique

Points for practice

1. If the patient is very thin or cachexic, the same gauge needle is used but it is not inserted so deeply. Using a smaller gauge needle requires more pressure to inject the liquid, which causes more discomfort, not less (King 2003).

2. Each Trust will have its own drug administration policy, which will indicate whether two nurses are required to check certain drugs. It will also indicate the role of the student nurse in drug administration.

3. When mixing the medicine, keep the needle inside the ampoule so that it remains sterile. If there is pressure within the vial, you may need to keep your thumb on the plunger. Mix gently as vigorous shaking will make it frothy and difficult to withdraw into the syringe.

4. Resheathing the needle *before* administration to the patient using the non-touch technique shown is perfectly safe and ensures that droplets of the drug are not inhaled or sprayed onto the skin as air is expelled from the syringe.

5. The recommended sites for intramuscular injection are the ventrogluteal aspect of the gluteus maximus and the lateral aspect of the vastus lateralis, which is one of the quadriceps (Greenway 2004, Nisbet 2006).
   If the patient is obese (i.e. has large amounts of adipose tissue) it is harder to be confident of intramuscular injection in the gluteus maximus and so the

vastus lateralis may be a better site (Nisbet 2006). Smaller intramuscular injections, such as vaccinations, are usually given into the deltoid area (see Figure 7.7).

6. The skin should be washed if visibly dirty. Some local policies no longer recommend skin cleansing prior to intramuscular injection because they regard it as unnecessary if the skin is clean (Wynaden et al 2005).

7. Leaving a little of the needle exposed means that it will be possible to remove the needle in the event of needle breakage.

8. If blood appears in the syringe at step 18, stop, withdraw the needle and start the procedure again with a new syringe and drug (Wynaden et al 2005). This happens only very rarely.

9. If you are unable to take the sharps bin to the patient, the needle and syringe should be placed in a cardboard tray or receiver and then tipped into the sharps bin without further handling (see page 249).

INTRAVENOUS DRUG ADMINISTRATION

Preparation

Patient

- Explain the procedure, to gain consent and co-operation.
- The patient should be resting in a chair or in bed.
- If the cannula site is covered by a bandage, this must be removed to allow inspection of the site.

Equipment/Environment

- Prescription chart and prescribed medicines.
- Syringes, needles and diluents as appropriate.
- 0.9% sodium chloride to flush the cannula **PFP1**.
- Alcohol-impregnated swab.
- Sharps bin.

Nurse

- **Only registered nurses who have undergone the appropriate training may administer intravenous medicines** in accordance with local policies **PFP2**.
- Wash and dry hands thoroughly. Additional protective clothing may be necessary if indicated by the patient's condition (see Chapter 9).
- Gloves and goggles may be necessary with certain medicines, e.g. cytotoxic drugs.

Procedure

1. Check the medicine as described on page 139. Whether you need to check these with another nurse will depend on the local intravenous drug administration policy **PFP2**.

2. Prepare the medicine for administration, as described for intramuscular injections (see page 150). Prepare 10 ml of 0.9% sodium chloride flush (more if several medicines are to be administered) **PFP1**.

3. At the bedside, check the medicine and the patient's nameband against the prescription again.

4. Adopt a comfortable posture (sitting is probably best) in a position that allows easy access to the cannula. Face the patient so that any adverse reaction may be observed, and if the patient is undergoing cardiac monitoring, this should also be in view.

5. Check the cannula site for signs of infection, phlebitis or discomfort/pain. If the site is bandaged, the bandage must be removed to allow inspection of the site. If there is an infusion running, the intravenous bolus may be administered via the small injection port that is situated approximately 10 cm from the end of the administration set. If this is used, the infusion must be stopped while the bolus is administered as described below, and then recommenced at the prescribed rate **PFP3**.

6. Thoroughly disinfect the rubber membrane of the injection port or injectable cap/bung according to local policy **PFP4**.

7. Before administering the medicine, administer a small amount (1–2 ml) of the 0.9% sodium chloride flush to confirm the patency of the cannula. If

resistance is felt, do not continue as this may dislodge a clot at the end of the cannula **PFP5**.

8. Slowly administer the medicine according to the prescription, the manufacturer's instructions, and/or local policies and procedures, using a needle-free system **PFP6** or small (25G) needle through an injectable rubber cap or port. If an infusional in progress is running, inject it through the injection port that is incorporated into the administration set (Figure 7.9).

9. Administer the remaining flush or, if a number of medicines are being given, flush between each one to prevent mixing in the cannula.

10. **Do not resheathe the needle.** Discard it, still attached to the syringe, into the sharps bin **PFP7**.

Post procedure

Patient	Equipment/Environment	Nurse
• Ensure the patient is comfortable. • Advise the patient to report any side effects.	• Dispose of needles, glass ampoules, etc., immediately into a sharps bin.	• Remove any protective clothing and wash hands. • Document the drug administration according to local policies and procedures. • Observe the patient for the desired effect and any adverse/side effects.

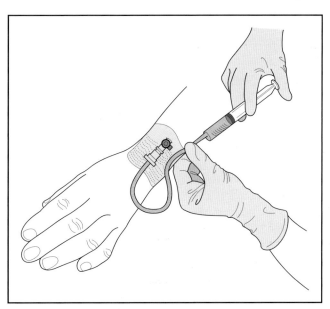

Figure 7.9 Intravenous injection technique

Points for practice

1. 0.9% sodium chloride is used for flushing purposes except in a few instances when the drug being administered is incompatible with sodium chloride. In these cases (e.g. amphotericin), 5% glucose should be used instead. In many NHS Trusts, the 0.9% sodium chloride or 5% glucose flush may be administered without prescription.

2. Although single-nurse administration is common for other routes of administration, some local policies require two nurses to administer intravenous drugs. It is vital that both nurses check thoroughly – you should never rely on the other nurse to check that it is correct.

3. If the infusion is prescribed to run at a very slow rate (e.g. dobutamine) it is better to use a separate cannula for bolus intravenous medications. If this is not possible, administer the flush and the bolus at a slower rate than the infusion to ensure that the infusion is not given faster than the prescribed rate.

4. Although some cannulae have an integral injection port, this should not be used for drug administration as it is difficult to keep the port clean and provides a reservoir for bacterial contamination.

5. If the patient complains of pain at the site, this may be due to infiltration or extravasation. If a small amount of flush solution is administered before the medicine to test patency, it will only be 0.9% sodium chloride rather than some potentially more damaging substance that is administered into the surrounding tissues.

6. There are a number of 'needle-free' injection caps available. These allow the syringe to be fitted directly into the injection cap without the need for a needle, thus reducing the risk of a needle-stick injury.

7. If you are unable to take the sharps bin to the patient, the needle and syringe should be placed in a cardboard tray or receiver and then tipped into the sharps bin without further handling (see page 249).

INSTILLATION OF NOSE DROPS

Preparation

Patient	Equipment/Environment	Nurse
• Explain the procedure, to gain consent and co-operation. PFP1.	• Prescription chart.	• **Only registered nurses may administer medicines** PFP2.
	• Nose drops as prescribed.	
• Ask the patient to lie down or sit in a chair where they will be able to hyperextend their neck. A pillow under the shoulders is beneficial.	• Clean tissues.	• Wash and dry hands thoroughly.
		• Additional protective clothing may be necessary if indicated by the patient's condition (see Chapter 9).

Procedure

1. Check the drops against the prescription chart (see page 139) noting whether the drops are to be instilled into one or both nostrils.
2. Ask the patient to hyperextend their neck.
3. Remove the cap from the nose drops container.
4. Using the dropper, administer the correct number of drops into each nostril, taking care not to touch the nose with the dropper PFP3.
5. Ask the patient to remain in this position for at least 2 minutes to allow absorption of the medication.
6. Wipe away any excess medication with a tissue.

Post procedure

Patient	Equipment/Environment	Nurse
• Ensure the patient is comfortable PFP4.	• Discard any used tissues into the clinical waste.	• Wash and dry hands thoroughly.
• Ask the patient to refrain from blowing their nose for 20 minutes following the procedure if possible.	• Return the nose drops to the correct storage area.	• Record administration on the prescription chart.
		• Evaluate the effect of the nose drops and document in the nursing records if appropriate.
		• Report any abnormalities.

Points for practice

1. Patients may be able to administer nose drops themselves. Nurses should ensure that they are using the correct procedure (see self-administration of medicines, page 135)

2. **Only registered nurses may administer medications.** Student nurses may only participate in the administration of nose drops under the direct supervision of a registered nurse. A registered nurse must countersign all student signatures.

3. It may be necessary to clean the nasal passages before administration of nose drops. This can be achieved by asking the patient to blow their nose or by using gauze moistened with 0.9% sodium chloride or water.

4. The nurse should explain that nose drops may run into the back of the throat, causing the patient to experience an unusual taste.

INSTILLATION OF EAR DROPS

Preparation

Patient	Equipment/Environment	Nurse
• Explain the procedure, to gain consent and co-operation.	• Prescription chart.	• **Only registered nurses may administer medicines** PFP3.
• Explain the action of the ear drops and the expected outcome.	• Ear drops as prescribed PFP2.	• Wash and dry hands thoroughly.
• Ask the patient to sit upright with their head tilted slightly away from the affected ear or to lie on their side with the affected ear uppermost PFP1.	• Clean tissues.	• Additional protective clothing may be necessary if indicated by the patient's condition (see Chapter 9).

Procedure

1. Check the ear drops against the prescription chart, noting which ear is to have the drops instilled (see page 139).
2. Remove the cap from the ear drops container.
3. Gently pull the pinna of the ear upwards and backwards.
4. Squeeze the bottle or dropper to dispense the prescribed number of drops into the ear taking care not to touch the skin with the dropper.
5. Release the pinna.
6. Replace the cap.
7. Instruct the patient to remain in this position for 1–2 minutes to allow the drops to reach the eardrum.
8. When the patient is sitting upright, use the tissue to wipe away any excess fluid from the outer ear.
9. If prescribed, repeat the process in the other ear after 5–10 minutes.

Post procedure

Patient	Equipment/Environment	Nurse
• Ensure the patient is comfortable.	• Store the ear drops in the appropriate place.	• Wash and dry hands thoroughly.
	• Dispose of clinical waste appropriately.	• Record administration on the prescription chart.
		• Evaluate the effect of the ear drops and document in the nursing records if appropriate.
		• Report any abnormalities.

Points for practice

1. Patients may be able to administer ear drops themselves. Nurses should ensure that they are using the correct procedure (see Self-administration of medicines, page 135).

2. If drops are prescribed for both ears there may be a separate bottle for each ear.

3. Only registered nurses may administer medications. Student nurses may only participate in the administration of ear drops under the direct supervision of a registered nurse. A registered nurse must countersign student signatures.

INSTILLATION OF EYE DROPS OR OINTMENT

Preparation

Patient	Equipment/Environment	Nurse
• Explain the procedure, to gain consent and co-operation.	• Prescription chart.	• **Only registered nurses may administer medicines** `PFP3`.
• Instruct the patient to tilt their head backwards and look up `PFP1`.	• Eye drops and/or ointment as prescribed `PFP2`.	• Wash and dry hands thoroughly.
• Explain that vision may be blurred for a short while after administration of the drops/ointment.	• Clean tissues.	• Additional protective clothing may be necessary if indicated by the patient's condition (see Chapter 9).

Procedure

1. Check the eye drops against the prescription, noting which eye is to have the drops/ointment instilled `PFP4`.
2. Remove the cap from the drops/ointment container.
3. Using your forefinger, gently pull the lower lid downwards to form a small pocket for the drops/ointment.
4. Hold the tissue beneath the eye.
5. Hold the dispenser between your thumb and forefinger about 2–3 cm from the patient's eye.
6. **Eye drops** – squeeze one drop into the eye and ask the patient to gently close the eye before the next drop. Repeat until the prescribed number of drops has been administered (Figure 7.10A).
   Eye ointment – squeeze the tube gently until a small amount (about 1–2 cm) of ointment forms a 'ribbon'. Apply the ribbon inside the lid margin, from the inner to outer aspect of the eye (Figure 7.10B). Do not touch any part of the eye with the tube.
7. Ask the patient to close (but not squeeze) their eyes to disperse the medication. They should keep their eyes closed for approximately 60 seconds.
8. Wipe away any excess medication that runs down the cheek with a clean tissue.
9. Replace the cap.
10. If more than one medication is required, repeat the process after 2–3 minutes.

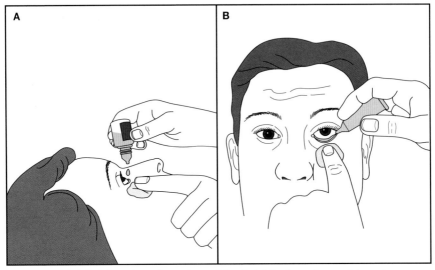

Figure 7.10 (A) Administration of eye drops, (B) administration of eye ointment

Post procedure

Patient	Equipment/Environment	Nurse
• Ensure the patient is comfortable and that vision has returned to normal.	• Store the eye drops/ointment in the appropriate place (eye drops may be kept in the refrigerator once opened). • Discard tissues into clinical waste.	• Wash and dry hands thoroughly. • Record administration on the prescription chart. • Evaluate the effect of the eye drops/ointment and document in the nursing records if appropriate. • Report any abnormalities.

Points for practice

1. Patients may be able to administer eye drops themselves. Nurses should ensure that they are using the correct procedure (see Self-administration of medicines, page 135). They may find it easier to self-administer the drops if they balance the bottle across the bridge of their nose and then squeeze the bottle to administer the drops.

2. If both eyes are being treated, there may be a separate bottle/tube for each eye. If one eye has obvious infection, treat that eye after the clean eye.

3. **Only registered nurses may administer medications**. Student nurses may only participate in the administration of eye drops/ointment under the direct supervision of a registered nurse. A registered nurse must countersign all student signatures.

4. If both eye drops and eye ointment are to be administered, administer the eye drops first as the grease base of the ointment can inhibit the absorption of drops.

TOPICAL APPLICATION

Preparation

Patient	Equipment/Environment	Nurse
• Explain the procedure, to gain co-operation and consent.	• Ensure the screens are pulled round to promote dignity and comfort.	• **Only registered nurses may administer medicines** PFP1.
• If possible patients should apply the cream or ointment themselves. The nurse should ensure they are applying it correctly (see Self-administration of medicines, page 135).	• Prescription chart. • Cream, ointment, lotion or topical patch as prescribed. • Gloves and sterile gauze to apply cream/lotion/ointment.	• Wash and dry hands thoroughly. • Put on gloves and apron. Gloves do not have to be sterile.

Procedure

1. Check the medicine against the prescription chart (see page 139 for checking procedure).
2. Locate the appropriate part of the body. If a topical patch is used, remove backing and apply the patch to clean, dry skin. If cream, ointment or lotion, rub in with a piece of sterile gauze, wearing gloves to avoid absorption of the active ingredients PFP2.

Post procedure

Patient	Equipment/Environment	Nurse
• Ensure the patient is comfortable.	• Remove apron and discard gloves and gauze in clinical waste.	• Wash and dry hands thoroughly. • Document that medicine has been administered and note condition of skin.

Points for practice

1. **Only registered nurses may administer medications**. Student nurses may only participate in the administration of topical applications under the direct supervision of a registered nurse. A registered nurse must countersign all student signatures.
2. If the medicine comes in the form of a topical patch, the site of application should be varied according to the manufacturer's instructions, i.e. the same site should not be used on consecutive applications and the patch may need to be removed after a certain time period.

VAGINAL PREPARATIONS

Preparation

Patient	Equipment/Environment	Nurse
• Explain the procedure, to gain co-operation and consent.	• Ensure the screens are pulled round to promote dignity and comfort.	• **Only registered nurses may administer medicines PFP1.**
• Wherever possible the woman should be assisted as necessary to administer the cream or pessary herself. If this is not possible, ask/assist her to lie on her back with her heels together, knees bent and legs apart.	• Prescription chart.	• Wash and dry hands thoroughly.
	• Cream or pessary as prescribed.	• Put on gloves and apron. Additional protective clothing may be necessary if indicated by the patient's condition (see Chapter 9).
	• Vaginal applicator.	
	• Gauze swabs or tissues.	
	• Protective pad or panty liner.	

Procedure

1. Check the medicine against the prescription chart (see page 139 for checking procedure).
2. Remove the pessary from the packaging and insert into the applicator. If using a vaginal cream, this is usually pre-loaded in the applicator.
3. Locate the vagina and gently insert the applicator as far as is comfortable.
4. Press the plunger to release the pessary or cream high in the vagina (Figure 7.11).
5. Remove the applicator and wipe away any traces of cream.

Post procedure

Patient	Equipment/Environment	Nurse
• Ensure patient is comfortable and has a panty liner or pad to protect their underwear.	• Discard vaginal applicator in clinical waste.	• Remove gloves and apron.
• Ask patient to remain recumbent for as long as possible PFP2.		• Wash and dry hands thoroughly.
		• Document that medicine has been administered.

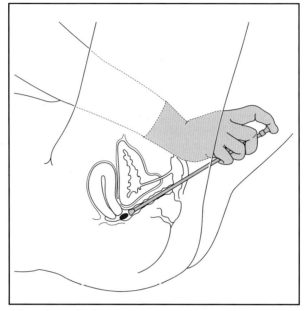

Figure 7.11 Insertion of a vaginal pessary

Points for practice

1. **Only registered nurses may administer medications**. Student nurses may only participate in the administration of vaginal preparations under the direct supervision of a registered nurse. A registered nurse must countersign student signatures. A male nurse will require a female chaperone to carry out this procedure.

2. Vaginal preparations are best administered last thing at night, when the patient will be recumbent for several hours, to allow absorption of the medication.

ADMINISTRATION OF SUPPOSITORIES

Preparation

Patient	Equipment/Environment	Nurse
• Explain the procedure, to gain consent and co-operation.	• Prescription chart.	• **Only registered nurses may administer medicines** PFP2.
• If the suppository is for drug administration (e.g. paracetamol) the bowels should be opened prior to administration if possible.	• Suppositories as prescribed PFP1.	
	• Cardboard tray or receiver.	• Wash and dry hands thoroughly. Put on apron and gloves.
	• Lubricant.	
• Draw the screens and ensure warmth and privacy.	• Gauze swabs or tissues.	• Additional protective clothing may be necessary if indicated by the patient's condition (see Chapter 9).
• Ask/assist patient to remove clothing below the waist, and lie in the left lateral position.		
• Place an absorbent pad under the buttocks.		

Procedure

1. Remove packaging around suppository.
2. Squeeze some lubricant onto a piece of gauze and lubricate the suppository.
3. Warn the patient that he/she will feel suppository being inserted into the rectum.
4. Ask patient to relax; encouraging deep breathing may help.
5. With your left hand, part the buttocks and inspect the anal area so as to avoid skin tags, haemorrhoids, etc. PFP3.
6. Gently insert the suppository into the anal canal blunt end first, using the index finger of your right hand (Figure 7.12) PFP4.
7. Repeat the process if more than one suppository is required.
8. Wipe away excess traces of lubricant from the anal area and remove gloves.
9. If it is an evacuant suppository (e.g. glycerine or bisacodyl) leave the patient in a comfortable position with a call bell at hand. To be effective, the suppositories should remain in position for at least 15 minutes and patients should be discouraged from opening their bowels before this time.
10. If the suppository is for drug administration (e.g. paracetamol) the patient should defaecate prior to administration if possible. This suppository is designed to be absorbed through the rectal wall and so the patient should be discouraged from opening their bowels for at least 30 minutes.

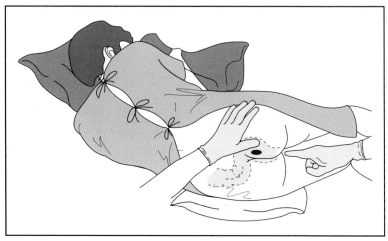

Figure 7.12 Administration of suppositories

Post procedure

Patient	Equipment/Environment	Nurse
• If the patient is unable to use the lavatory, assist them to use a bedpan/ commode as necessary. • Offer a bowl of water to wash hands.	• Dispose of waste and equipment appropriately.	• Remove apron and wash hands. • Note bowel action following the suppository and document/report result.

Points for practice

1. If the suppository is for drug administration, this must be prescribed and checked as described on page 139. If medication per rectum may be required whilst a patient is in theatre, it is good practice to ask the patient to sign a consent form for this prior to surgery.

2. **Only registered nurses may administer medications**. Student nurses may only participate in the administration of suppositories under the direct supervision of a registered nurse. A registered nurse must countersign all student signatures.

3. It is necessary for the patient to be in the left lateral position because of the position of the rectum. This means that for effective insertion, even left-handed nurses must use their right hand to insert the suppository.

4. There is evidence to suggest that if the suppository is inserted blunt end first, insertion and retention of the suppository is easier (Moppett 2000).

RESPIRATORY ROUTE – METERED DOSE INHALER

Preparation

Patient	Equipment/Environment	Nurse
• Explain the procedure, to gain co-operation and consent.	• Metered dose inhaler and any adjuncts such as a volumatic spacer **PFP1**.	• **Only registered nurses may administer medicines** **PFP2**.
• Patients should use inhalers themselves, the nurse's role is to ensure they utilise the correct technique (see page 135).	• Prescription chart.	• Hands should be clean.

Procedure

1. Check the inhaler against the prescription chart (see page 139 for procedure).

   Using inhaler only:
   Instruct patient to remove cap and shake inhaler. They should then breathe out gently and make a seal around the mouthpiece (Figure 7.13). As they start to inhale, they should press the canister and hold their breath for a minimum of 10 seconds and then exhale gently. Instruct the patient to wait 30 seconds before taking another inhalation.

   Using inhaler with volumatic spacer:
   Instruct the patient to shake the inhaler and insert it into the spacer (see Figure 7.14). They place their mouth around the mouthpiece and press the canister once to release the drug into the spacer. Instruct the patient to breathe in and out slowly five times and then remove the spacer from the mouth. The patient should wait 30 seconds before administering a second dose.

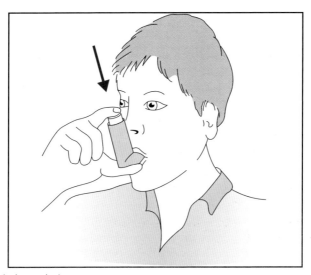

Figure 7.13 Inhaler technique

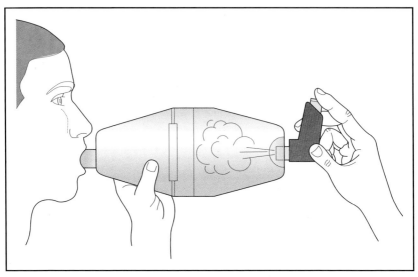

Figure 7.14 Volumatic spacer device

Post procedure

Patient	Equipment/Environment	Nurse
• Ensure the patient is comfortable.	• Replace the cap and place the inhaler in patient's medicine cupboard or lock in drug trolley.	• Document that medicine has been administered and evaluate effectiveness.
• If the inhaler contains steroids the mouth should be rinsed with water or a mouthwash following administration **PFP3**.	• Spacers should be taken apart and washed in clean water approximately once a month **PFP4**.	

Points for practice

1. Adjuncts such as a volumatic spacer device can be used for patients who are very breathless or find it difficult to co-ordinate pressing the canister and breathing (see Figure 7.14). It also helps to reduce deposition of the powder in the throat, which can lead to hoarseness and loss of voice (Esmond 2001). Specialist respiratory nurses will be able to advise on other suitable inhaler devices should the patient have difficulty using a metered dose inhaler.

2. **Only registered nurses may administer medications**. Student nurses may only participate in the administration of inhaled medications under the direct supervision of a registered nurse. A registered nurse must countersign student signatures.

3. Rinsing the mouth after inhalation of steroids reduces deposition of the powder in the mouth, which can lead to candida (thrush) infections.

4. Spacers should be replaced every 6–12 months as the volumatic valve wears out.

References and further reading

British National Formulary (BNF). BMJ Publishing Group Ltd., Royal Pharmaceutical Society of Great Britain and RCPCH Publications, London.

This is published twice a year and so the most recent edition should be used. This publication lists all medications and their classification. It identifies indications, cautions, contraindications and dose for each medication.

Best C. (2005) Caring for the patient with a nasogastric tube. *Nursing Standard* **20**(3):59–65.

This is a comprehensive article covering all the major aspects relating to insertion and management of a nasogastric tube, including the administration of medicines via the nasogastric tube.

Cannaby AM, Evans L, Freeman A. (2002) Nursing care of patients with nasogastric feeding tubes. *British Journal of Nursing* **11**:366–372.

The article includes a useful literature review of the management of NG tubes. It addresses: types of tubes, tube placement and checking procedures, feeding rest periods, drug administration, blocked tubes and flushing techniques, and syringe sizes. They then surveyed Nutrition Nurse Specialists to discuss the practices that they recommend.

Court S, Lamb B. (1997) *Childhood and adolescent diabetes*. John Wiley & Sons, Chichester.

The chapter on insulin strategies (Chapter 11) discusses injection sites, injection techniques and factors that can affect absorption. Although the focus is on childhood and adolescents the information is equally relevant to adult patients and clients.

Deeks PA, Byatt K. (2000) Are patients who self-administer their medicines in hospital more satisfied with their care? *Journal of Advanced Nursing* **13**(2):395–400.

An interesting survey of 202 patients who were being discharged home from two general medical wards in a hospital in Central England. The article provides some useful background information about self-administration of medicines and the perceived benefits. The survey found that the majority of patients under the age of 60 years would prefer to self administer their own medications and that those who were able to do so were more likely to report their overall care as excellent and were more satisfied with the discharge process.

Department of Health. (2007) *Safer management of controlled drugs: A guide to good practice in secondary care (England)*. DH: London.

This sets out systems for procuring, storing, supplying, transporting, prescribing, administering, recording and safely disposing of CDs whilst ensuring that patients who require CDs have appropriate and convenient access. The document is organised in chapters dealing with legislative requirements and guiding principles.

Dimond B. (2003) Law relating to the classification and regulation of controlled drugs. *British Journal of Nursing* **12**(8):502–504.

A useful article relating the legal aspects of controlled drugs.

Esmond G (ed). (2001) *Respiratory Nursing*. Baillière Tindall, Edinburgh, in association with the Royal College of Nursing, London.

This is an excellent book on all aspects of respiratory nursing. Chapter 5 describes the different types of inhalers available and how each should be used.

Greenway K. (2004) Using the ventrogluteal site for intramuscular injection. *Nursing Standard* **18**(25):39–42.

This article discusses the use of the ventrogluteal site for intramuscular injection in place of the dorsogluteal (upper, out quadrant of the buttock) that was traditionally used. Includes the rationale for use of this site, clear diagrams to locate the ventrogluteal site and discusses potential complications when using the dorsogluteal site.

Griffith R, Griffiths H, Jordan S. (2003) Administration of medicines part 1: the law and nursing. *Nursing Standard* **18**(2):47–54.

A useful article in relation to the law and the nurse. It has an interesting section on risk management.

King L. (2003) Subcutaneous insulin injection technique. *Nursing Standard* **17**(34):45–52.

This article discusses the injection technique required to ensure insulin in not inadvertently injected into muscle. It discusses the rationale for the 'pinch up' method, which reduces the risk of inadvertent intramuscular injection by lifting the subcutaneous tissue away from the muscle.

Lapham R, Agar H. (2003) *Drug calculations for nurses: a step-by-step guide*. Hodder Arnold, London.

A useful book that covers the many different types of drug calculations that nurses are likely to use in clinical practice. There are plenty of exercises so that you can test how good you are!

Little K. (2000) Skin preparation for intramuscular injections. *Nursing Times* **96**(46): NTPlus:86.

This article reviews the evidence available to support skin preparation practice and found that there is little reliable evidence to support or discontinue the practice of cleansing the skin with alcohol prior to intramuscular injection. She argues that skin preparation should continue as a sensible precaution to protect patients from the admittedly small but significant risk of soft-tissue infection.

Marsden J. (2003) Correct administration of topical eye treatment. *Nursing Standard* **17**(30):42–44.

A useful article that discusses the principles of administration and the rationale for the procedure in relation to different ophthalmic problems.

Moppett S. (2000) Which way is up for a suppository? *Nursing Times* **96**(19):NTPlus: 12–13.

This article discusses the rationale relating to the most effective way to insert a suppository (blunt end first) in order to aid retention.

Nisbet AC. (2006) Intramuscular gluteal injections in the increasingly obese population: retrospective study. *BMJ* **332**:637–638.

A study to measure the ventrogluteal depth of 100 patients. The conclusion was that standard green and blue needles do not reach the gluteal muscle in a considerable number of patients, which results in the injection being given subcutaneously instead of intramuscularly. It recommends that the vastus lateralis muscle may be a better choice in obese patients.

Nursing and Midwifery Council. (2004) *Guidelines for the administration of medicines*. NMC, London.

These guidelines give an overview of the principles of administration that should be followed. They are regularly reviewed so it is important to check the NMC website (www.nmc-uk.org) to check you have the latest guidelines.

Nursing and Midwifery Council. (2006) *A-Z advice sheet: Medicines management*. NMC, London.

The NMC gives comprehensive advice regarding the administration of medicines and associated issues such as whether to crush medication and covert administration of medication.

Small PS. (2004) Preventing sciatic nerve injury from intramuscular injections; literature review. *Journal of Advanced Nursing* **47**(3):287–296.

A review of the literature surrounding intramuscular injection techniques and an interesting summary of the legal cases as a result of sciatic nerve injury. There is wide agreement that the ventrogluteal site is preferable to reduce the risk of accidental injury to the sciatic nerve. She argues that if the dorsogluteal site is chosen the nurse must fully appreciate the anatomy of the site and potential risk of damage to the sciatic nerve.

Wynaden D, Landsborough I, Chapman R, McGowan S, Lapsley J, Finn M. (2005) Establishing best practice guidelines for administration of intramuscular injections in the adult: a systematic review of the literature. *Contemporary Nurse* **20**:267–277.

This Australian paper presents a comprehensive review of approximately 150 articles in order to produce these best practice guidelines. The guidelines address all aspects of intramuscular injection including: choice of site, needle size, volume of medication, techniques to reduce discomfort, skin cleansing and angle, and speed of injection.

Websites

http://www.asthma.org.uk

This site has animations showing how to use several inhaler and spacer devices.

www.bnf.org

On-line BNF has a version of the latest edition available. In order to access this registration is required, but there is no charge for this.

www.testandcalc.com

This is a commercial site to which you can subscribe. However, it also has several free tests that you can access and mark on line. There are sections that show how to work out the answers if you have problems.

Notes

8

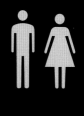

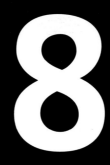

Elimination

OBSERVATION OF FAECES

Principles

Normal faeces (also known as a 'stool') is brown, soft and formed; it has an odour, but should not be offensive smelling. When observing faeces, the following should be noted and any abnormality reported:

- Amount – particularly if diarrhoea, as patients may lose a lot of fluid this way.
- Frequency – the 'normal' frequency will vary from patient to patient.
- Consistency – the normal consistency is soft and formed. The following should be noted: hard faeces (constipation); liquid (diarrhoea); mucus evident (ulcerative colitis or Crohn's disease); fatty, offensive smelling and floats (steatorrhoea, seen in biliary disease); whether parasites are present.
- Colour – a pale, putty colour suggests the absence of bile pigments. The presence of bright-red blood may indicate bleeding from haemorrhoids or rectal bleeding. If the stool appears black and tarry in consistency (melaena), this indicates digested blood from the stomach or small intestine. If the stool is black and hard in consistency, this may be the result of iron medication.
- Pain/discomfort associated with a bowel action.
- Flatus – the presence of this indicates gut motility and is an important observation following abdominal surgery.

OBTAINING A SPECIMEN OF FAECES

Preparation

Patient	Equipment/Environment	Nurse
• Explain the procedure, to gain consent and co-operation.	• Sterile stool specimen container with spatula. • Specimen bag. • Completed pathology request form, e.g. microbiology.	• Put on apron and gloves. • Additional protective clothing may be necessary if indicated by the patient's condition (see Chapter 9).

Procedure

1. Ask/assist the patient to use a bedpan or commode (see pages 183–185).
2. Open the sterile specimen container and remove the spatula (usually attached to the lid of the container) **PFP1**.
3. Use the spatula to remove a small quantity of faeces from the bedpan. Place the faeces and the spatula in the container and secure the lid.
4. Complete the patient's details on the label of the container. If a series of specimens is being collected, ensure the correct sequence is identified.
5. Place the specimen container in the specimen bag, seal it and insert the pathology request form into the pocket **PFP2**.

Post procedure

Patient	Equipment/Environment	Nurse
• Ensure the patient is comfortable. • Offer/assist with hand washing.	• Dispose of faeces and place bedpan in the washer or disposal system as appropriate. • Clean the commode, if used, according to local policy. • Place specimen in the designated area to await transport to the laboratory.	• Remove gloves and apron and wash hands. • Document that specimen has been collected.

Points for practice

1. If no spatula is provided, use a disposable wooden tongue depressor.
2. Occasionally, testing for occult blood is done on the ward. The manufacturer's instructions should be followed.

ADMINISTRATION OF AN ENEMA

Preparation

Patient	Equipment/Environment	Nurse
• Explain the procedure, to gain consent and co-operation.	• Prescription chart **PFP2**.	• Put on apron and gloves.
• Draw screens to ensure privacy.	• Enema as prescribed (Figure 8.1) **PFP3**.	• Additional protective clothing may be necessary if indicated by the patient's condition (see Chapter 9).
• Ask/assist the patient to remove clothing below the waist and lie in the left lateral position **PFP1**.	• Cardboard tray/receiver.	
	• Gauze swabs/tissues.	
	• Lubricant.	
• Cover the patient with a blanket.	• Bedpan or commode, plus toilet paper.	
• Place an absorbent pad under the buttocks.		

Procedure

1. Check the anal area for soreness, haemorrhoids or skin tags. If present seek advice before proceeding.
2. Remove the cover or removable tip from the nozzle (Figure 8.1) and lubricate the tip.
3. Ask the patient to relax and take deep breaths.

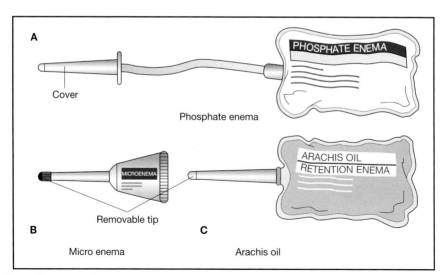

A

Cover

Phosphate enema

PHOSPHATE ENEMA

MICROENEMA

ARACHIS OIL
RETENTION ENEMA

Removable tip

B

Micro enema

C

Arachis oil

Figure 8.1 Types of enema

4. Part the buttocks with the left hand. With the right hand, hold the nozzle of the enema and *gently* insert it through the anus and into the anal canal PFP4.

5. Squeeze the bag/pack until all the contents have been deposited – the bag/pack may be rolled (like a tube of toothpaste) to expel the last of the contents (Figure 8.2).

6. While still squeezing and keeping the bag rolled, gently withdraw the nozzle PFP5.

7. Wipe away any residual lubricant and leave the patient dry. Cover the patient.

8. **Evacuant enema**: ask the patient to hold the enema for as long as possible but the effect is likely to be rapid. Assist the patient onto the bedpan or commode as necessary (see pages 183–185).

   Retention enema (drug administration): the patient should be instructed to stay in the left lateral position for at least 30 minutes to aid retention and absorption of the fluid. Raising the foot of the bed may also help.

Post procedure

Patient	Equipment/Environment	Nurse
• The patient may feel faint and/or nauseous. • Offer a bowl of water to wash hands after using the bedpan/commode.	• Dispose of clinical waste appropriately.	• Remove gloves and apron. • Wash hands. • Document/report the result of the enema.

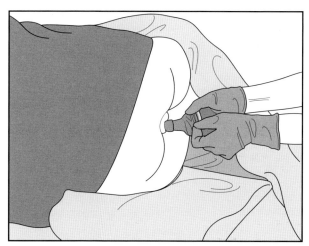

Figure 8.2 Administering an enema

Points for practice

1. It is necessary for the patient to be in the left lateral position because of the position of the rectum.

2. If the enema is for drug administration, this must be prescribed and checked as described on page 139.

3. Some enemas may need to be warmed before administration. Do this by placing in warm water.

4. For effective administration, even left-handed nurses must use their right hand to insert the nozzle of the enema.

5. Keeping the bag rolled while removing the nozzle on completion of the enema prevents fluid running back into the bag.

ASSISTING WITH A BEDPAN

Preparation

Patient	Equipment/Environment	Nurse
• Assess the patient to determine the type of bedpan required – standard or slipper type **PFP1**. • Ensure privacy and dignity are maintained throughout.	• Bedpan and cover. • Toilet paper.	• An apron should be worn. Gloves should be worn when handling the bedpan and assisting with toileting. • Additional protective clothing may be necessary if indicated by the patient's condition (see Chapter 9). • Dependent patients may require two nurses for this procedure.

Procedure

1. Take the covered bedpan and toilet paper to the bedside.
2. Ensure the screens are completely drawn.
3. Raise the bed to a safe working height (see Chapter 13 Moving and handling).
4. Ask/assist the patient to raise their buttocks and place the bedpan underneath the patient's pelvis – wide rim of bedpan under the buttocks, and narrow area between legs (Figure 8.3).
5. When using a slipper bedpan (Figure 8.4), if the patient cannot raise their buttocks assist the patient to roll to one side and slip the bedpan underneath from the side; talcum powder applied to the bedpan will assist this process if the patient is sweating. The handle end should be positioned towards the legs.
6. For female patients, make sure that the legs are slightly apart, otherwise urine may trickle down the legs onto the sheet. For male patients, ensure that the penis is positioned over the bedpan **PFP2**.
7. Preserve the patient's privacy and dignity by covering the patient with the bedclothes.
8. Ensure the call bell is within easy reach and leave the patient but remain within earshot.
9. When the patient has finished, provide assistance with cleansing as necessary and remove the bedpan.
10. If the patient has had a bowel action the perianal area should be washed with soap and water and dried thoroughly.

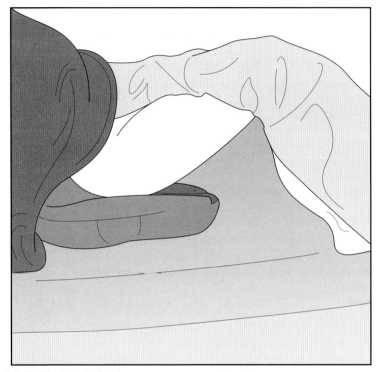

Figure 8.3 Positioning the bedpan

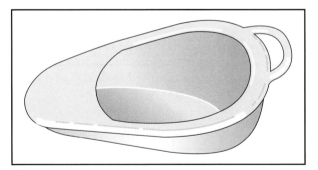

Figure 8.4 The slipper bedpan

Post procedure

Patient	Equipment/Environment	Nurse
• Ensure patient comfort – straighten the sheets, rearrange pillows, bedclothes, etc., as necessary.	• Measure urine if necessary.	• Remove gloves and apron and wash hands.
	• Dispose of excreta safely and place the bedpan in the washer or disposal system as appropriate.	• Record urine output and/ or bowel action as appropriate.
• Offer the patient a bowl of water to wash hands.	• Return the bedside table and belongings to within easy reach of patient.	

Points for practice

1. The slipper bedpan (Figure 8.4) is used for patients who are unable to sit on a standard bedpan (Figure 8.3). Its wedge shape makes it easier to insert and more comfortable to use. It is inserted with the handle under the patient's legs and the smooth, flat part underneath the buttocks.

2. When using a slipper bedpan male patients may find it easier to use a urinal as well (see page 188).

ASSISTING WITH A COMMODE

Preparation

Patient	Equipment/Environment	Nurse
• Explain the procedure, to gain consent and co-operation.	• Clear the bed area and draw the screens to ensure privacy.	• An apron should be worn. Gloves should be worn when assisting with toileting and removing the commode.
• Assess the patient's level of mobility and ability to assist with the procedure.	• Commode containing clean bedpan.	• Additional protective clothing may be necessary if indicated by the patient's condition (see Chapter 9).
	• Toilet paper.	

Procedure

1. Take the commode (with seat in place, covering bedpan) and toilet paper to the bedside **PFP1**.
2. Ensure the screens are completely drawn.
3. Check the bed brakes are on.
4. Position the commode so that the patient has sufficient room to get out of bed without banging their legs, and apply the brakes.
5. Assist the patient to a sitting position on the edge of the bed.
6. Adjust the bed to enable the patient to stand easily.
7. Offer slippers and dressing gown.
8. Assist the patient as necessary to transfer to the commode.
9. If the patient is frail, position the commode so that the patient is close to and facing the bed. Apply the brakes and place a pillow at the edge of the bed for the patient to lean on (Figure 8.5).
10. Ensure the patient has access to a call bell. Provide privacy by leaving but remain within earshot.
11. When the patient has finished, assist with cleaning/washing as necessary.

Post procedure

Patient	Equipment/Environment	Nurse
• Assist the patient back to bed and offer a hand wash.	• Measure urine if required.	• Remove gloves and apron and wash hands.
• Rearrange pillows, bedclothes, bedside table, etc., as necessary.	• Dispose of excreta safely and place the bedpan in the washer or disposal system as appropriate.	• Record urine output and/or bowel action as appropriate.
	• Clean the commode according to local policy **PFP2**.	

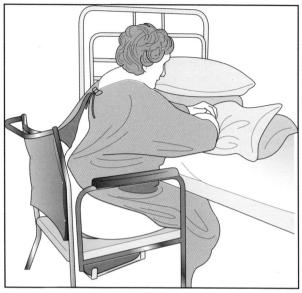

Figure 8.5 Frail patient using commode

Points for practice

1. Placing the toilet roll in a small bowl or receiver will prevent it rolling off the commode when being wheeled to the bedside.

2. Local policy for cleaning the commode may vary but cleaning with hot water with detergent followed by thorough drying is sufficient. The use of detergent is important as it breaks up grease and improves the ability of water so that approximately 80% of micro-organisms are removed (Wilson 2006).

USE OF URINAL

Preparation

Patient	Equipment/Environment	Nurse
• Explain the procedure, to gain consent and co-operation.	• Urinal and cover **PFP1**.	• An apron and gloves should be worn.
• Assess the patient's level of mobility and ability to assist with the procedure.	• Provide privacy.	• Additional protective clothing may be necessary if indicated by the patient's condition (see Chapter 9).

Procedure

1. Ask/assist the patient to adopt an appropriate position. Standing is best if this is possible **PFP2**.
2. If necessary, assist the patient to hold the urinal and position the penis inside.
3. When the patient has finished urinating, assist as necessary with clothing and returning to bed/chair.
4. Cover the urinal and take to the sluice/dirty utility room.

Post procedure

Patient	Equipment/Environment	Nurse
• Offer the patient hand washing facilities.	• Measure urine if appropriate and then dispose of safely unless being collected, e.g. 24-hour urine collection (see page 203).	• Remove gloves and apron and wash hands.
	• Discard the urinal or clean it as per local policy.	• Record amount on fluid balance chart (where applicable) (see page 190).

Points for practice

1. Many patients prefer to keep a urinal at the bedside. This should be kept in a holder attached to the bed, not on the bedside locker or bed table.
2. If the patient is sitting on the edge of the bed, make sure the brakes are on and the bed is at a suitable height for their feet to touch the floor.

MONITORING FLUID BALANCE

Preparation

Patient	Equipment/Environment	Nurse
• Explain any activities that may be required of the patient.	• Fluid balance chart. • Measuring jug.	• Gloves should be worn when handling body fluids. • Additional protective clothing may be necessary if indicated by the patient's condition (see Chapter 9).

Procedure

1. All oral, intravenous and nasogastric intake should be recorded on the fluid intake side of the fluid balance chart (**Figure** 8.6). If continuous bladder irrigation is in progress, this should also be recorded. If a separate chart is used for continuous bladder irrigation then the urine output must be transposed to the fluid balance chart.

2. Record on the output section all urine output, diarrhoea or stoma output, nasogastric aspiration and vomit. Any other output that can be measured or weighed (e.g. wound drainage) should also be recorded.

3. The sections labelled 'Other' should be annotated according to individual patient requirements (see **Figure** 8.6).

4. Patients who are independent in meeting their oral needs should be asked to note the nature and quantity of their oral fluid intake. If the patient is not independent, the nurse must do this.

5. Patients who are independent in meeting elimination needs will often be able to measure and chart their own urine output. If they are unable to do this themselves, provide them with a clearly labelled jug to leave in the sluice/toilet area.

6. Assess individual needs and monitor and record input and output at regular intervals.

7. A new chart will be needed for each 24-hour period. The fluid intake and output for the previous day is then totalled and the balance is calculated

Fluid balance chart

Hospital/Ward:	ST. SWITHINS		Date: 01.01.08

Hospital number: **1234567**

Surname: **SMITH**	Forenames: **FRANK**

Date of birth: **01.01.1949**	Sex: **MALE**

	Fluid intake				Fluid output			
Time (hrs)	Oral	IV	Other (specify route)	Urine	Vomit	Other (specify)		
01.00	NBM	B/F 500				WOUND DRAIN		
02.00		N/SALINE 0.9%						
03.00								
04.00								
05.00		↓						
06.00		5% Dex		400	90			
07.00		1000						
08.00								
09.00	↓							
10.00	30 water							
11.00	30 water							
12.00	30 water			500				
13.00	30 water							
14.00	30 water							
15.00	30 water							
16.00	30 water							
17.00	30 water	↓						
18.00	60 water	5% Dex		450				
19.00	60 water	500						
20.00	60 water							
21.00	60 water							
22.00	100 TEA							
23.00								
24.00		↓		350	50			
TOTAL	580ml	2000		1700	140			

KEY:
NBM = NIL BY MOUTH
B/F = BROUGHT FORWARD

ALL MEASURMENTS IN MILLILITRES (ML.)
TOTAL INPUT   =   580 + 2000 = 2580 ML.
TOTAL OUTPUT = 1700 + 140   = 1840 ML.
                            BALANCE = +740 ML.

Figure 8.6 Example of fluid balance chart

Points for practice

1. If the patient is on a fluid restriction (e.g. in renal failure), all oral fluid – including, for example, any milk with cereal – has to be recorded.

2. Accurate recording of intake and output is vital to be able to calculate the fluid balance. Gaps in recording (e.g. if the patient has been to theatre or for a test) make the balance inaccurate. In acute situations it may be necessary to measure the urine output every hour.

3. If there is more intake than output, the patient is in a positive fluid balance. If there is more output than intake, the patient is in a negative fluid balance.

4. In some patients, especially renal patients who do not pass urine, fluid balance is monitored by weighing the patient. Changes in weight will reflect fluid loss or gain.

APPLICATION OF A PENILE SHEATH

Preparation

Patient	Equipment/Environment	Nurse
• Explain the procedure to gain consent and co-operation.	• Sheath sizing tool and correctly sized penile sheath `PFP1`.	• Hands must be clean and an apron and gloves should be worn.
• Ensure complete privacy and dignity.	• Card or tissue paper with a hole cut `PFP2`.	• Additional protective clothing may be necessary if indicated by the patient's condition (see Chapter 9).
	• Catheter drainage bag or leg bag as appropriate.	
	• Warm water, soap, disposable washcloth and towel.	

Procedure

1. Assist the patient into a supine position.

2. Prepare the catheter drainage bag.

3. Expose the patient's genitalia and place the penis gently on a towel. Measure the penis and select the correct size sheath `PFP3`.

4. Gently grasp the shaft of the penis. If the patient has not been circumcised, retract the foreskin.

5. Wash the tip of the penis at the urethral meatus and work outwards.

6. Wash the shaft of the penis in a downward stroke.

7. Repeat until the penis is clean, then rinse and dry gently. Leave to air dry for a few minutes.

8. If using a skin protection wipe, allow to dry according to manufacturer's instructions before applying the sheath. Do not use powders or creams as it will affect adhesion.

9. Ensure the foreskin is returned to its normal position.

10. Clip hair at the base of the penis if this is likely to prevent the adhesive sticking `PFP4`.

11. Place the penis through the hole cut in the card or tissue paper `PFP2`. Gently press on the pubic hairs to keep them out of the way of the adhesive during application.

12. Apply the sheath according to the manufacturer's guidelines (Figure 8.7). Application will differ depending on whether you are using a one-piece or two-piece sheath `PFP5`.

13. If using a leg bag, attach it to the leg first to avoid sheath twisting.

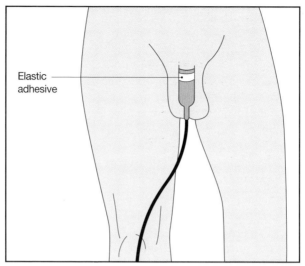

Elastic
adhesive

Figure 8.7 Penile sheath in position

Post procedure

Patient	Equipment/Environment	Nurse
• Ensure patient is comfortable.	• Dispose of clinical waste appropriately.	• Remove gloves and apron and wash hands.
• Advise the patient to wearing loose clothing and underwear.	• Observe for leakage from the bag/tubing.	• Document application of sheath, noting the condition of the penile skin.
• Readjust clothing/ bedclothes as necessary.		• Check skin integrity at least once daily when attending to patient hygiene `PFP6`.

Points for practice

1. The correct sizing of a penile sheath is important as if it is too small there may be difficulties with fitting and it may restrict urinary flow and blood to the penis. If it is too loose, it will crease and leakages will occur.

2. A card or tissue paper with a hole for the penis acts as pubic hair protector. Some companies provide sheath packages, which include a pubic hair shield (Robinson 2006a).

3. Sizing tools for correct selection of penile sheath come as either a tape measure or a card with cut-out sections in various sizes. If using a cut-out it must be measured with the cut-out section on the upper surface of the penis and not underneath. Always use the sizing tool supplied by the same company as the penile sheath as companies use different measuring scales (Robinson

2006a). Measurement should be taken from the shaft of a flaccid penis, just behind the glans. It the penis is erect then the circumference should be measured and the penile sheath also fitted in this state. Penile retraction (penis disappears into the pelvic cavity), is not uncommon in older men and its extent must be determined before attempting to attach a sheath and a shorter than normal sheath may be used. However, if complete retraction is evident when the patient is sitting down a penile sheath is not appropriate as it may not stay in position, and will roll off as the penis retracts causing disconnection and leakage.

4. It is important that hair is clipped rather than shaved as this could make the skin sore.

5. Penile sheaths are available in latex and non-latex (silicone) materials, can be one-piece or two-piece, are available in short and standard lengths, have various penile shaft fittings and have anti-kinking devices (Booth & Lee 2005). Sheaths in silicone materials are recommended because of the risk of latex allergy. One-piece sheaths have adhesive already applied to the inside of the sheath. Fitting instructions do vary; therefore, it is important to carefully follow the manufacturer's instructions. Two-piece sheaths come with a double-sided hydrocolloid strip. One side of the strip adheres to the penis shaft and the other to the sheath. The adhesive strip should be gently stretched and then attached to the shaft of the penis beginning from behind the glans in a spiral direction. Ensure the sides meet. The sheath is then rolled over the shaft of the penis adhering to the outer side of the strip (Robinson 2006a).

6. Skin soreness or breakdown on the shaft of the penis can be caused by poor hygiene, pulling or rough handling of the sheath and latex allergies. If the skin on or around the penis becomes damaged, use of a sheath should not be continued until healing has taken place.

OBSERVATION OF URINE

Preparation

Patient	Equipment/Environment	Nurse
• Explain the procedure to gain co-operation and consent.	• Clean container/jug for the urine.	• An apron should be worn. • Additional protective clothing may be necessary if indicated by the patient's condition (see Chapter 9).

Procedure

1. Ask the patient to provide a urine sample.
2. If necessary, transfer the specimen to a clear container or jug **PFP1**.
3. Observe the urine for colour, concentration, odour and the presence of particles **PFP2**.

Post procedure

Patient	Equipment/Environment	Nurse
• Answer any questions.	• Dispose of urine safely. • Clean or dispose of the container/jug according to local policy.	• Document urine observation and report any abnormalities.

Points for practice

1. A clear container or jug should be used if possible to enable the colour and clarity of the urine (e.g. presence of particles) to be assessed.
2. Dark-yellow urine indicates that it is more concentrated than normal. The smell of ammonia will develop if the urine specimen is left standing. A malodorous or 'fishy' smell and/or particles in the urine may indicate a urine infection. Any blood in the urine should always be reported, although if the patient is a woman, menstruation may be the cause.

URINALYSIS

Preparation

Patient	Equipment/Environment	Nurse
• Ask the patient to provide a urine specimen, or obtain a specimen, e.g. catheter specimen (see page 201).	• Fresh urine specimen in clean container/jug **PFP1**. • Urine reagent sticks. • Watch with a second-hand.	• An apron and gloves should be worn. • Additional protective clothing may be necessary if indicated by the patient's condition (see Chapter 9).

Procedure

1. Check the expiry date of the reagent sticks and make sure that you are familiar with the manufacturer's instructions for use.

2. Remove a stick, making sure that you do not touch the coloured reagent pads with your hands. Replace the lid **PFP2**.

3. Dip the stick into the urine so that the reagent pads are completely covered. Remove straight away and tap the stick against the side of the container/jug to remove excess urine **PFP3**.

4. Note the time on your watch. Accurate timing is crucial.

5. When the correct period of time has elapsed, read off the results by holding the stick alongside (but not touching) the pot and comparing the colour of each reagent pad with those displayed on the side (**Figure 8.8**). Make a mental note of the results **PFP4**.

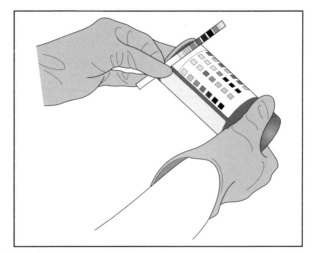

Figure 8.8 Urine testing

Urine reagent sticks commonly test for the following:

- Specific gravity (SG – normal range 1001–1035). A raised SG may indicate concentrated urine due to dehydration; a low SG may indicate renal disease or diabetes insipidus (Rigby & Gray 2006).
- pH (normal range 4.5–8.0). Normal urine is slightly acidic; a low pH may indicate respiratory or metabolic acidosis and a high pH may indicate respiratory or metabolic alkalosis. Some drugs can affect the urinary pH: ascorbic acid can make the urine more acidic and sodium bicarbonate, potassium citrate and sodium citrate can make the urine more alkaline (Skinner 2005).
- Protein, glucose, ketones, blood and bilirubin. All of these are negative in normal urine. The presence of these abnormalities might indicate the following (Rigby & Gray 2006):
  - Protein (proteinuria) – urinary tract infection, pyelonephritis, pre-eclampsia, congestive cardiac failure.
  - Glucose (glycosuria) – diabetes mellitus, acute pancreatitis, Cushing's syndrome or sometimes in pregnancy.
  - Ketones (ketonuria) – excessive fat metabolism due to diabetic ketoacidosis, vomiting or severe dieting/starvation.
  - Blood (haematuria) – kidney disorders (e.g. glomerulonephritis), disorders of the urinary tract (e.g. kidney stones, tumours, infection), trauma or menstruation.
  - Bilirubin – liver disease (e.g. hepatitis) or biliary tract obstruction (e.g. gall stones, carcinoma of the head of pancreas).

Post procedure

Patient	Equipment/Environment	Nurse
• Discuss the result with the patient as appropriate.	• Discard the used stick in the clinical waste and dispose of the urine safely. • Clean or dispose of the container/jug according to local policy.	• Remove gloves and apron and wash hands. • Document urinalysis and report any abnormalities.

Points for practice

1. The urine sample should be fresh as urine left to stand will become alkaline (Skiner 2005).
2. The lid of the reagent-sticks pot must always be replaced immediately after use to prevent moisture getting in.

3. Removing excess urine from the testing stick will prevent it dripping onto the bottle and prevent the coloured reagent pads running into each other, which could give inaccurate readings.

4. Make a mental note of the results or if necessary jot them down on a piece of paper. Do not take the patient's charts into the sluice/dirty utility room to prevent contamination or splashing with water.

MIDSTREAM SPECIMEN OF URINE

Preparation

Patient	Equipment/Environment	Nurse
• Explain the procedure, to gain consent and co-operation. • Ensure privacy and dignity are maintained.	• Toilet, urinal or bedpan. • Sterile universal specimen pot. • Gauze swabs, soap and water. • Paper towels.	• Apron and gloves should be worn. • If assisting the patient, additional protective clothing may be necessary if indicated by the patient's condition (see Chapter 9).

Procedure

Male patient

1. Instruct/assist the patient to retract the foreskin and clean the skin surrounding the urethral meatus with soap and water, using each gauze swab only once. Dry with paper towels.

2. Ask the patient to start urinating into the urinal/toilet then stop, pass the middle part of the stream into the specimen pot (10 ml is sufficient) and then finish urinating into the urinal/toilet **PFP1**.

Female patient

1. Instruct/assist the patient to clean the urethral meatus with soap and water, using each gauze swab only once. Swab from front to back. Dry with paper towels.

2. Ask the patient to start urinating into the urinal/toilet then stop, pass the middle part of the stream into the specimen pot (10 ml is sufficient) and then finish urinating into the urinal/toilet **PFP1**.

Post procedure

Patient	Equipment/Environment	Nurse
• Offer the patient hand washing facilities. • Ensure the patient is comfortable.	• Discard all waste appropriately.	• Ensure the specimen pot is securely closed. • Remove gloves and wash hands. • Complete patient details on the label **PFP2**. Place in a plastic specimen bag with the pathology request form (Figure 8.9) **PFP3**. • Place the specimen in the refrigerator for dispatch to the laboratory as soon as possible **PFP4**. • Document the date and time of specimen collection in the patient records.

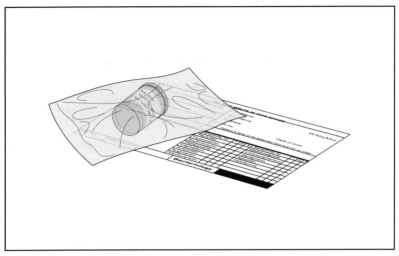

Figure 8.9 Urine specimen and request form

Points for practice

1. Some specimen pots for midstream urine sample have a special funnel attached to facilitate collection. This is removed and discarded before the specimen is sent to the laboratory.

2. The patient's details should include: surname, first name, date of birth, hospital number, ward and type of specimen (i.e. MSU).

3. If the test is ordered by computer, the request form should be printed off to accompany the sample.

4. The specimen should be placed in a refrigerator because urine readily supports growth of bacteria. The multiplication of bacteria in specimens stored at room temperature can give misleading results (Wilson 2006).

CATHETER SPECIMEN OF URINE

Preparation

Patient

- Explain the procedure, to gain consent and co-operation.
- Maintain dignity and privacy throughout the procedure.

Equipment/Environment

- Alcohol-impregnated swab.
- Non-toothed clamp **PFP1**.
- A 20 ml syringe **PFP2**.
- Sterile universal specimen container.

Nurse

- Hands must be washed and dried thoroughly.
- An apron and gloves should be worn.
- Additional protective clothing may be necessary if indicated by the patient's condition (see Chapter 9).

Procedure

1. If there is no urine present in the catheter tubing, clamp it below the sampling port for 15–20 minutes to allow urine to collect.
2. Clean the sampling port on the tubing with the alcohol-impregnated swab and allow it to dry.
3. Insert the syringe into the sampling port and aspirate the required amount of urine **PFP3**. If a needle is being used, take care not to go right through the tubing and out the other side (Figure 8.10).
4. Transfer the urine to the specimen pot and replace the lid securely **PFP4**.
5. Remove the clamp, if used, to allow free drainage.

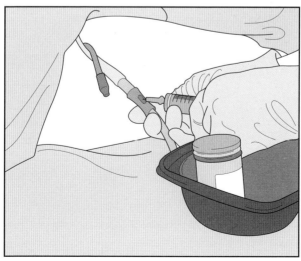

Figure 8.10 Obtaining catheter specimen of urine

Post procedure

Patient	Equipment/Environment	Nurse
• Ensure the patient is comfortable.	• Discard clinical waste and sharps appropriately.	• Remove gloves and apron and wash hands.
		• Label the specimen **PFP5** and place it in a plastic specimen bag with the laboratory request form (**Figure 8.9**) **PFP6**.
		• Place the specimen in the refrigerator for dispatch to the laboratory as soon as possible **PFP7**.
		• Document the date and time of specimen collection in the patient's records.

Points for practice

1. It is important that a non-toothed clamp is used to prevent damage to the tubing.
2. Some catheter bags have a 'needle-free' sampling port as part of the tubing, which allows the syringe to be connected without a needle. If a needle is required, an orange needle (25G) should be used.
3. A 10 ml sample of urine is usually sufficient.
4. If a needle has been used, remove it from the syringe before transferring the specimen, in case it falls into the pot and contaminates the specimen.
5. The patient's details should include: surname; first name; date of birth; hospital number; ward; and date, time and type of specimen (i.e. CSU).
6. If the test is ordered by computer, the request form should be printed off to accompany the sample.
7. The specimen should be placed in a refrigerator because urine readily supports growth of bacteria. The multiplication of bacteria in specimens stored at room temperature can give misleading results (Wilson 2006).

24-HOUR URINE COLLECTION

Preparation

Patient	Equipment/Environment	Nurse
• Explain the procedure, and assess the patient's ability to participate in obtaining the collection.	• Urinal/bedpan as required and jug. • A 24-hour urine collection container (more than one may be required) **PFP1**. • Bed/door sign indicating 24-hour urine collection is in progress, time started and when due to be completed.	• Apron and gloves should be worn. • Additional protective clothing may be necessary if indicated by the patient's condition (see Chapter 9).

Procedure

1. Label the container clearly with the patient's name, hospital number and ward.

2. When urine is passed, discard it. The 24-hour period begins at this point.

3. Every time the patient passes urine, it is collected and placed in the container, which is stored in the sluice/dirty utility room **PFP2**.

4. If the patient is undertaking collection independently, check compliance and continued understanding.

5. Ask/assist the patient to empty their bladder at the end of the 24-hour collection period.

Post procedure

Patient	Equipment/Environment	Nurse
• Advise the patient when the 24-hour period is completed.	• Remove sign from the bed/door. • Clean or discard the jug according to local policy.	• Record completion time of the 24-hour urine collection. • Ensure that the urine collection and laboratory request form are sent to the laboratory as soon as possible **PFP3**.

Points for practice

1. Bottles containing hydrochloric acid or nitric acid may be required if the collection is to test for: catecholamines, creatinine, calcium, phosphate, oxalate, citrate and magnesium. Plain bottles are usually required for: protein,

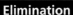

sodium, potassium, uric acid, cortisol, chloride and histamine. The volume of acid will need to be deducted from the total volume – check local policy.

2. Should a sample of urine become contaminated or accidentally be discarded, the collection must be terminated and restarted.

3. If the test is ordered by computer, the request form should be printed off to accompany the sample.

EARLY MORNING URINE SPECIMEN

Preparation

Patient	Equipment/Environment	Nurse
• Provide a clear explanation of the collection procedure and the need for three consecutive early morning specimens `PFP1`. • Ensure privacy and dignity are maintained. • The urine specimen should be collected as soon as possible after waking.	• Sterile universal specimen pot. • Gauze swabs, soap and water. • Paper towels. • Toilet, urinal or bedpan.	• Apron and gloves should be worn if the patient requires assistance. • Additional protective clothing may be necessary if indicated by the patient's condition (see Chapter 9).

Procedure

1. Ask/assist female patients to clean and dry the vulval area around the urinary meatus, using wet gauze swabs and paper towels. Ask male patients to retract the foreskin and clean and dry the end of the penis.

For cytology

2. Ask/assist the patient to hold the specimen pot in a gloved hand and pass **the beginning and the end** of the stream of urine into the pot `PFP2`. The middle of the stream should be passed into the toilet, bedpan or urinal `PFP3`.

3. Repeat the procedure on the next two consecutive days if required.

For other test (e.g. TB, pregnancy)

2. Ask/assist the patient to hold the specimen pot in a gloved hand and pass the first part of the stream into the pot. The remainder of the stream should be passed into the toilet, urinal or bedpan.

Post procedure

Patient	Equipment/Environment	Nurse
• The patient may be unaware of the possible diagnosis; deal with the patient's questions with sensitivity.	• Ensure the specimen pot is securely closed. Label the pot `PFP4` and place in a plastic specimen bag with the laboratory request form. Refrigerate until dispatch to the laboratory `PFP5`.	• Document the date and time of specimen collection in the patient's records.

Points for practice

1. A urine specimen for cytology is requested when a malignancy is suspected. The patient may not be aware of this at this point and care must be taken to avoid unnecessary alarm.

2. The first part and end of the stream of urine are collected as these are most likely to contain malignant cells if present in the bladder.

3. If the patient is unable to stop and start the stream of urine, the bladder should be emptied completely into a sterile container and a small portion (10–20 ml) of that amount put into the specimen pot.

4. The patient's details should include: surname; first name; date of birth; hospital number and ward. Each specimen must also be clearly labelled with the date and time, and numbered 1, 2 or 3 to ensure the correct order is known in the laboratory.

5. If the test is ordered by computer, the request form should be printed off to accompany the sample.

FEMALE CATHETERISATION

Preparation

Patient

- Explain the procedure, to gain consent and co-operation.
- Ensure the patient's privacy and dignity are maintained throughout.
- Ask/assist the patient to wash the perineal area and dry thoroughly.

Equipment/Environment

- Clean trolley or other appropriate surface.
- Sterile catheterisation pack **PFP1**.
- Two urinary catheters of appropriate size **PFP2**.
- Sachet of sterile 0.9% sodium chloride.
- Catheter bag with stand/holder.
- Single use sterile anaesthetic lubricating gel.
- Sterile universal specimen container.
- A 10 ml syringe and 10 ml ampoule of sterile water for injection.
- Disposable waterproof absorbent pad.
- Alcohol hand-rub or hand washing facilities.
- Good light source.

Nurse

- Wash and dry hands thoroughly.
- An apron should be worn. Additional protective clothing may be necessary if indicated by the patient's condition (see Chapter 9).
- Two nurses may be necessary if the patient needs assistance to adopt the required position.

Procedure

1. Take the prepared trolley to the patient's bedside and position it on the right or left depending on the nurse's dominant hand.

2. Raise the bed to a safe working height and ensure a good light source.

3. Ask/assist the patient to adopt a supine position with knees flexed and thighs relaxed to externally rotate the hip joints. If the patient is unable to adopt this position, she can be assisted onto her side with her upper leg flexed at the hip and knee.

4. Arrange the bedclothes to expose the genital area, and place the disposable pad beneath the buttocks.

5. Wash your hands or clean them with alcohol hand-rub.

6. Ensuring principles of asepsis are maintained, open the catheterisation pack and any additional packs and equipment.

7. Open the catheter, but do not remove it from its internal wrapping, and place it in the sterile receiver on the trolley. Expose the tip of the catheter by pulling off the top of the wrapper at the serrated edge.

8. Pour the sachet of 0.9% sodium chloride into the gallipot.

9. Open the catheter bag and arrange it at the side of the bed, ensuring that the catheter connection is easily accessible and remains sterile.

10. Draw up the amount of sterile water required to inflate the balloon **PFP3**.

11. Attach the nozzle to the anaesthetic lubricating gel.

12. Wash your hands or clean them with alcohol-based rub, and put on the sterile gloves **PFP4**.

13. Place sterile dressing towels onto the bed area between the patient's legs and over the patient's thighs.

14. Using a gauze swab and your non-dominant hand, retract the labia minora to expose the urethral meatus (**Figure 8.11**). This hand should be used to maintain labial separation until catheterisation has been completed.

15. Clean the perineal area with 0.9% sodium chloride, using a new gauze swab for each stroke and cleaning from the front towards the anus.

16. Insert nozzle of the lubricating/anaesthetic gel into the urethra. Squeeze the gel into the urethra, remove and discard the tube. Leave for approximately 5 minutes **PFP5**.

17. Place the receiver holding the catheter on the sterile towel between the patient's legs.

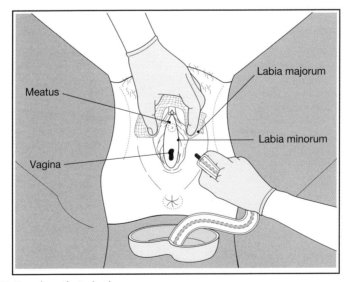

Figure 8.11 Female catheterisation

18. Holding the catheter so that the distal end remains in the receiver and gradually advancing it out of its wrapper, introduce the catheter into the urethra in an upward and backward direction for approximately 5–7 cm or until urine flows out of the catheter end. Advance the catheter a further 5 cm. Do not force the catheter PFP6.

19. Inflate the balloon with the correct amount of water (see **Figure 8.14**).

20. Place a small amount of urine (10–20 ml) into the specimen pot PFP7.

21. Attach the catheter drainage bag and position it so that there is no pulling on the catheter.

Post procedure

Patient	Equipment/Environment	Nurse
• Make sure the patient is dry and comfortable.	• Dispose of equipment and clinical waste appropriately.	• Remove gloves and apron and wash hands.
• If the patient's condition allows, encourage oral fluids PFP8.	• Measure and record the amount of urine contained in the receiver.	• Document catheterisation in the patient's records.
• Ensure the catheter drainage bag is positioned below the patient's bladder PFP9.	• Send the specimen, with the request form, to the laboratory as soon as possible, for culture and sensitivity.	• Monitor urine output as appropriate.

Points for practice

1. A catheterisation pack usually contains the following sterile items: kidney dish/receiver, dressing towels, gloves, gallipot and gauze swabs. If a catheterisation pack is not available, a sterile dressing pack containing gloves can be used and the other items added as required.

2. When choosing the size of catheter to be inserted, choose the smallest size possible. The external diameter of the catheter shaft is measured in Charrière (ch) also known as French gauge (Fg) units. For most women a 12 ch/Fg or 14 ch/Fg will be adequate, although a larger size may be necessary if there is blood or sediment in the urine. A second catheter is useful in case catheterisation is unsuccessful with the first. Female length catheters are 23–26 cm. They reduce the risk of kinking and looping, and so allow more efficient drainage, and can also be more easily concealed if being used with a leg bag (Robinson 2006b). However, they are not suitable for all women.

3. The volume of water required will be indicated on the catheter. A balloon size of 10 ml is recommended for the routine drainage of clear urine, as this is usually sufficient to retain the catheter. Larger balloon sizes may irritate the

bladder and cause bladder spasm and bypassing of urine. 30–80 ml balloons are used in specialised catheters in urology units and should not be used for routine catheterisation (Robinson 2004). It is important to use the exact amount of water as indicated on the catheter.

4. Concerns about contamination of the hands during urethral cleansing and instillation of gel can be overcome by using two pairs of sterile gloves (one on top of the other) at the start of the procedure. The outer pair can then be removed after cleansing, prior to catheter insertion.

5. Anaesthetic/lubricant gel is recommended for use in female catheterisation to prevent urethral trauma and to reduce discomfort for the patient (Pomfret 2004, Woodward 2005).

6. If the catheter is accidentally inserted into the vagina, leave it in place to prevent it happening again, and use a new catheter. Once this is successfully in place, remove the first catheter from the vagina.

7. Urine from the sterile receiver or contained within the plastic wrapper can be tipped into the specimen pot.

8. Traditionally people with an in-dwelling urinary catheter were encouraged to have a high fluid intake, which was thought to reduce the incidence of catheter-associated urinary-tract infections (CAUTI). This has now been discredited, but good fluid intake will result in more dilute urine, which in turn enables smaller diameter catheters to be used and so reduce the risk of urethritis (Pomfret 2006).

9. Positioning the catheter drainage bag below the level of the patient's bladder aids gravity flow and prevents reflux of urine. Ensure the bag is not touching the floor as this is an infection risk (Head 2006).

MALE CATHETERISATION

Preparation

Patient

- Explain the procedure, to gain consent and co-operation.
- Ensure the patient's privacy and dignity are maintained throughout.
- Ask/assist the patient to wash the penis and perineal area and dry thoroughly.

Equipment/Environment

- Clean trolley or other appropriate surface.
- Sterile catheterisation pack **PFP1**.
- Two urinary catheters of an appropriate size **PFP2**.
- Single use sterile anaesthetic lubricating gel.
- Sachet of sterile 0.9% sodium chloride.
- A 10 ml syringe and 10 ml ampoule of sterile water for injection.
- Catheter drainage bag and stand/holder.
- Sterile universal specimen container.
- Alcohol hand-rub or hand washing facilities.
- Waterproof absorbent pad.
- Good light source.

Nurse

- Wash and dry hands thoroughly.
- An apron should be worn. Additional protective clothing may be necessary if indicated by the patient's condition (see Chapter 9).
- Two nurses may be necessary if the patient needs assistance to adopt the required position **PFP3**.

Procedure

1. Take the prepared trolley to the patient's bedside and position it on the right or left depending on the nurse's dominant hand.

2. Raise the bed to a safe working height and ensure a good light source.

3. Ask/assist the patient to adopt a supine position with the legs extended.

4. Arrange the bedclothes to expose the genital area, and place the absorbent pad underneath the buttocks.

5. Wash your hands or clean them with alcohol hand-rub.

6. Ensuring the principles of asepsis are maintained, open the catheterisation pack and any additional packs and equipment.

7. Open the catheter, but do not remove it from its inner wrapper, and place it in the sterile receiver on the trolley. Expose the tip of the catheter by pulling off the top of the wrapper at the serrated edge. Replace it in the sterile receiver.

8. Pour the sachet of 0.9% sodium chloride into the gallipot.

9. Draw up the amount of sterile water required to inflate the balloon **PFP4**.

10. Open the catheter drainage bag and arrange it at the side of the bed, ensuring the attachment tip is easily accessible and remains sterile.

11. Wash your hands or clean them with alcohol hand-rub. Put on the sterile gloves **PFP5**.

12. Tear a hole in the centre of the sterile towel. Cover the patient's abdomen and thighs with the towel, with the penis protruding through the hole.

13. Attach the nozzle to the anaesthetic lubricating gel.

14. With your non-dominant hand and using a piece of sterile gauze, grasp the shaft of the penis and retract the foreskin.

15. Clean the glans penis with the sterile 0.9% sodium chloride, ensuring the tips of the fingers remain sterile (**Figure 8.12A**).

16. Still holding the penis, insert the nozzle of the anaesthetic lubricating gel into the urethra and instill the gel into the urethra (**Figure 8.12B**).

17. Massage the gel along the urethra and wait 5 minutes for it to act.

18. Place the receiver containing the catheter between the patient's thighs.

19. Grasp the shaft of the penis with your non-dominant hand and hold the penis upwards, to extend the peno-scrotal flexure **PFP6**.

20. With your dominant hand holding and gradually withdrawing the wrapper, insert the catheter 15–25 cm into the urethra until urine flows (**Figure 8.13**). If resistance is met at the external sphincter, extend the penis further towards the abdomen. Ask the patient to cough or strain gently as if passing urine. If resistance continues, do not force the catheter: stop the procedure and seek medical advice.

21. When urine is flowing, advance the catheter further, to ensure the catheter is in the bladder.

22. Inflate the balloon with the correct amount of sterile water (**Figure 8.14**).

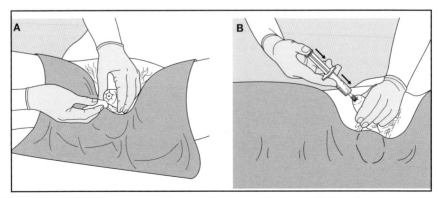

Figure 8.12 (A & B) Cleaning the glans penis and instilling anaesthetic gel

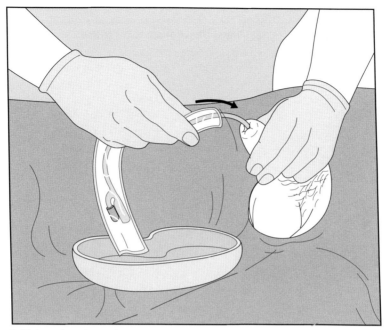

Figure 8.13 Inserting the catheter

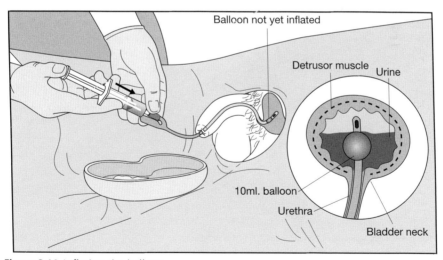

Figure 8.14 Inflating the balloon

23. Place a small amount of urine (10–20 ml) into the specimen pot PFP7.
24. Attach the catheter drainage bag and position it so that it is well supported to prevent traction on the catheter.
25. Ensure the foreskin is gently pushed back over the glans penis.

Post procedure

Patient

- Ensure the patient is dry and comfortable.
- If the patient's condition allows, encourage oral fluids PFP8.
- Ensure the catheter drainage bag is positioned below the patient's bladder PFP9.

Equipment/Environment

- Dispose of equipment and clinical waste appropriately.
- Measure and record the amount of urine contained in the receiver.
- Send the specimen and the request form to the laboratory as soon as possible, for culture and sensitivity testing.

Nurse

- Remove gloves and apron and wash hands.
- Record catheterisation in the patient's documentation.
- Monitor urine output as appropriate.

Points for practice

1. A catheterisation pack usually contains the following sterile items: kidney dish/receiver, dressing towels, gloves, gallipot and gauze swabs. If a catheterisation pack is not available, a sterile dressing pack containing gloves can be used and the other items added as required.

2. When choosing the size of catheter to be inserted, choose the smallest size possible. For most men a 12 ch/Fg or 14 ch/Fg will be adequate, although a larger size may be necessary if there is blood or sediment in the urine. Trauma from catheter insertion is commonly associated with urethral stricture formation. Trauma arises when too large a catheter is used, when the catheter is forced on insertion or when the balloon is inflated in the urethra. Necrosis in the bladder neck may also result from an overly large catheter or balloon. The standard length urinary catheter is better known as the male length catheter and ranges from 40 to 44 cm (Robinson 2006B). A second catheter is useful in case catheterisation is unsuccessful with the first.

3. In most hospitals, only registered nurses who have received additional training may perform male catheterisation (Doherty 2006).

4. The volume of water required will be indicated on the catheter. A balloon size of 10 ml is recommended for the routine drainage of clear urine, as this is usually sufficient to retain the catheter. Larger balloon sizes may irritate the bladder and cause bladder spasm and bypassing of urine. 30–80 ml balloons are used in specialised catheters in urology units and should not be used for routine catheterisation (Robinson 2004). It is important to use the exact amount of water indicated on the catheter.

5. Concerns about contamination of the hands during urethral cleansing and instillation of gel can be overcome by using two pairs of sterile gloves (one on top of the other) at the start of the procedure. The outer pair can then be removed after cleansing, prior to catheter insertion.

6. If difficulties are encountered force or pressure must not be used. Asking a male patient to cough may allow the catheter to more easily pass the prostate (Head 2006).

7. Urine from the sterile receiver or contained within the plastic wrapper can be tipped into the specimen pot.

8. Traditionally people with an in-dwelling urinary catheter were encouraged to have a high fluid intake, which was thought to reduce the incidence of catheter-associated urinary-tract infections (CAUTI). This has now been discredited, but good fluid intake will result in more dilute urine, which in turn enables smaller diameter catheters to be used and so reduce the risk of urethritis (Pomfret 2006).

9. Positioning the catheter drainage bag below the level of the patient's bladder aids gravity flow and prevents reflux or urine. Ensure the bag is not touching the floor as this is an infection risk (Head 2006).

URETHRAL CATHETER CARE

Preparation

Patient	Equipment/Environment	Nurse
• Explain the procedure, to gain consent and co-operation **PFP1**. • Ensure the patient's privacy and dignity are maintained. • Place the patient in a supine position with knees and hips flexed and slightly apart.	• Soap, water and disposable washcloth. • Clean towel.	• Wash and dry hands thoroughly. • Put on apron and gloves.

Procedure

Female patients

1. Clean the vulval area from above downward using warm soapy water **PFP2**.
2. Clean the catheter by gently wiping in one direction away from the catheter-meatal junction. Rinse well.
3. Dry the area by patting with a towel.

Male patients

1. Retract the foreskin before cleaning **PFP2**.
2. Clean the shaft of the catheter away from the catheter-meatal junction and rinse well.
3. Dry the area by patting with a towel.
4. Replace the foreskin on completion of cleaning.

Post procedure

Patient	Equipment/Environment	Nurse
• Ensure the patient is dry and comfortable.	• Dispose of all waste appropriately.	• Remove gloves and apron and wash hands. • Record catheter care and report any abnormalities.

Points for practice

1. Where possible, patients should be taught to attend to their own meatal and perineal hygiene, thus reducing the risk of cross-infection. Powders or lotions should not be used after cleansing as these trap organisms in the area.

2. The main aim of cleansing is to remove secretions and encrustation. Cleansing with soap and water has been shown to be as effective as any other method. There is no evidence of reduction in bacteria if antimicrobial/antiseptic agents are used (Pomfret 2006). Cleaning in addition to normal hygiene practice is not necessary and daily bathing or showering is sufficient to maintain meatal hygiene unless there is excessive exudate or encrustation (Pomfret 2006).

Note: Supra-pubic catheters are inserted through the abdominal wall, directly into the bladder. The insertion site should be treated as a surgical wound (see page 258).

EMPTYING A CATHETER BAG

Preparation

Patient	Equipment/Environment	Nurse
• Explain the procedure to the patient, although it should not cause any discomfort.	• Measuring jug **PFP1** and paper towel to cover.	• Wash and dry hands thoroughly.
• The patient may prefer the bed to be screened.	• Alcohol-impregnated swabs.	• Gloves and an apron should be worn.
		• Additional protective clothing may be necessary if indicated by the patient's condition (see Chapter 9).

Procedure

1. Take the covered jug and other equipment to the bedside.

2. If the drainage bag is on a floor stand, it does not need to be removed from the stand for emptying. If the bag is hanging on the side of the bed, it may need to be removed from its holder. Hold the bag over the jug, making sure that the drainage port does not touch the jug (Figure 8.15).

3. Open the drainage port and allow the urine to flow into the jug. Close the drainage port.

4. Wipe the outlet tap again with a new alcohol-impregnated swab.

5. Reposition the catheter bag as necessary to ensure that the drainage port is not touching the floor and the tubing is not kinked, to allow free drainage into the bag.

6. Cover the jug and take it to the sluice. Measure the amount of urine and discard **PFP2**.

Post procedure

Patient	Equipment/Environment	Nurse
• If the patient's condition allows, encourage oral fluids.	• Clean or discard the urine jug according to local policy **PFP3**.	• Remove gloves and apron and wash hands.
		• Record amount on fluid balance chart if appropriate.

Points for practice

1. The container used to collect the drained urine will vary according to local policy; it may be single use or one that is disinfected after each use. If using a disinfected jug it should be one that is only used for urine. This should be a different colour or design from those used for drinking water.

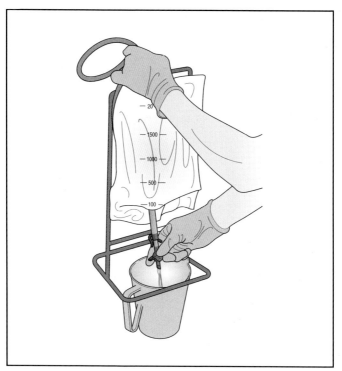

Figure 8.15 Emptying the catheter bag

2. If hourly urine measurement is required, a special drainage bag is used which incorporates a small reservoir that can be emptied into the drainage bag without opening the 'closed' system (Figure 8.16).

3. The cleaning of the jug will vary according to local policy. If disposable, it will be discarded. If not disposable, it may be disinfected, or placed in a bedpan washer or returned to the sterile supplies department for decontamination.

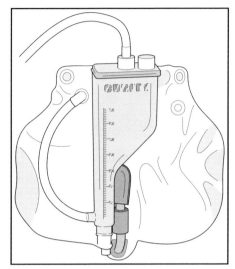

Figure 8.16 Hourly measurement catheter bag

CONTINUOUS BLADDER IRRIGATION

Preparation

Patient

- Explain the procedure, to gain consent and co-operation.
- Ensure the patient's privacy and dignity are maintained.
- The patient will be catheterised with a three-way urethral catheter.

Equipment/Environment

- Clean trolley or other appropriate surface.
- Sterile dressing pack containing gloves.
- Sterile dressing towel.
- Antiseptic skin-cleansing solution according to local policy.
- Non-toothed clamp.
- Sterile jug.
- Sterile 'Y' shaped irrigation set and fluid as prescribed (usually 0.9% sodium chloride) at room temperature PFP1.
- Infusion stand PFP2.
- Large catheter drainage bag.
- Alcohol hand-rub.

Nurse

- Wash and dry hands thoroughly.
- An apron should be worn.
- Additional protective clothing may be necessary if indicated by the patient's condition (see Chapter 9).

Procedure

1. Take the trolley and equipment to the bedside.
2. Open the irrigation fluid bags and hang on the infusion stand.
3. Maintaining asepsis, attach and prime the irrigation set to expel all air. Close the flow control clamp of the irrigation set PFP3.
4. Ask/assist the patient to adopt a supine position, and expose the catheter and catheter drainage tube.
5. Clamp the catheter using a non-toothed clamp or the clamp on the catheter-bag tubing (Figure 8.17) PFP4.
6. Wash and dry your hands.
7. Maintaining asepsis, open the dressing pack and other equipment, attach the disposal bag to the side of the trolley and pour antiseptic solution into the gallipot.
8. Cleanse your hands with alcohol hand-rub, allow to dry and then put on the sterile gloves.

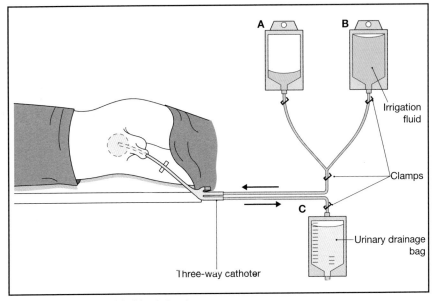

Figure 8.17 Continuous bladder irrigation

9. Place the sterile towel underneath the irrigation inlet of the catheter.

10. Cover both the catheter and spigot with sterile gauze, and touching only the gauze, remove the spigot from the irrigation port of the catheter and discard.

11. Thoroughly clean around the irrigation port with antiseptic solution, using each swab only once and wiping in the same direction.

12. Maintaining asepsis, attach the irrigation set to the irrigation port, but do not open the flow control clamp.

13. Release the clamp on the catheter and allow accumulated urine to drain. Empty the contents of the catheter bag into the sterile jug (see page 218).

14. Discard gloves.

15. Open the flow control clamp and set irrigation at the prescribed rate, ensuring that fluid/urine is draining freely into the catheter bag **PFP5** (Figure 8.17).

Post procedure

Patient	Equipment/Environment	Nurse
• Assist the patient into a comfortable position.	• Dispose of equipment and waste appropriately.	• Remove apron and wash hands.
• Advise the patient to report any bladder distension, pain or discomfort **PFP6**.	• Measure the volume of urine and discard.	• Record the time of commencement and the volume of irrigation fluid being infused on the fluid balance chart.
		• Check the volume in the catheter drainage bag at least every hour for the first 24 hours, empty as necessary and record on fluid balance chart **PFP7**.

Points for practice

1. 3 l bags of irrigation solution are preferable, as they require less frequent changing and interruption of the closed system. This reduces the risk of infection.

2. Irrigation fluid should be suspended from a separate infusion stand from that used for intravenous infusions.

3. When priming the irrigation set, make sure that only one clamp (e.g. A or B, Figure 8.17) is open. This will prevent irrigation fluid running from one bottle to the other (Scholtes 2002).

4. It is important to use a non-toothed clamp to prevent damage to the tubing.

5. The rate of infusion will vary according to the degree of haematuria (blood in the urine). The aim is to obtain drainage fluid that is rosé in colour. Haematuria will be greatest in the first 12 hours following surgery and 6–9 l of irrigation fluid is likely to be required. This should fall to 3–6 l in the second 12 hours. Only one bag of irrigation fluid is used at a time. When the first bag is empty the second bag can be commenced immediately ensuring continuous flow. In the meantime, the empty bag can be replaced (Selfe 2006).

6. If clot retention is suspected (the output stops and the patient complains of pain and discomfort) irrigation should be stopped immediately and the problem reported. A bladder washout may be required (see page 225).

7. The volume of irrigation fluid being infused and the amount of drainage in the catheter bag should be recorded on a fluid balance chart. The difference between the two figures is the urine output (Table 8.1).

Table 8.1 Example of irrigation-fluid and urine-output charting

Time	Input (irrigation fluid)			Total output (irrigation fluid plus urine)	Total output (running total)	Urine (total output minus input)	Urine (running total)
	A	B					
0600	3000			600	600		
0630				750	1350		
0700				700	2050		
0730				750	2800		
0800		3000		500	3300	300	300
0830				750			
0900				750			
0930				800			
1000	3000			850	3150	150	450
1030				800			
1100				750			
1130				800			
1200				850	3200	200	650

BLADDER WASHOUT/LAVAGE

Preparation

Patient	Equipment/Environment	Nurse
• Explain the procedure, to gain consent and co-operation **PFP1**. • Ensuring dignity and privacy are maintained, position the patient to allow access to the catheter. • An absorbent, waterproof pad should be placed under the patient's buttocks.	• Clean trolley or other appropriate surface. • Sterile dressing pack containing gloves. • Sterile dressing towel. • A 50 ml or 60 ml bladder tip syringe **PFP2**. • Sterile jug. • Sterile washout solution as prescribed (most commonly 0.9% sodium chloride) at room temperature **PFP3**. • Two sterile bowls or receivers. • Antiseptic cleansing solution according to local policy. • Alcohol hand-rub or hand washing facilities. • Non-toothed clamp. • Sterile spigot if washout solution is to be retained. • New catheter drainage bag.	• Wash and dry hands thoroughly. • An apron should be worn. • Additional protective clothing may be necessary if indicated by the patient's condition (see Chapter 9).

Procedure

1. Take the prepared trolley to the patient's bedside and position it on the right or left depending on the nurse's dominant hand.

2. Maintaining asepsis, open the sterile dressing pack and additional equipment including the sterile jug, bladder syringe and sterile bowls/receivers. Pour antiseptic solution into the gallipot. Pour washout solution into the jug.

3. Open the catheter drainage bag and place it in an accessible position, leaving the cover on the catheter connector to maintain sterility.

4. Arrange the bedclothes to expose the genital area and check the absorbent pad is under the buttocks.

5. Wash and dry your hands or clean them using alcohol hand-rub, and put on the sterile gloves.

6. Draw up 30–40 ml of washout fluid into the syringe (note the amount) and expel the air.

7. Place the sterile towel between the patient's legs, creating a sterile field.

8. Place one receiver on the sterile towel.

9. Clamp the catheter.

10. Cover both the catheter and drainage tube with sterile gauze, and touching only the gauze, disconnect the catheter from the tubing. Place the end of the catheter in the sterile receiver.

11. Clean the end of the catheter with antiseptic solution and attach the bladder syringe. Unclamp the catheter and gently instil the solution into the bladder (Figure 8.18).

12. Remove the syringe and allow the solution to drain out naturally into the second sterile receiver. If the solution does not drain, aspirate gently using the bladder syringe **PFP4**. Repeat the process, using 30–40 ml of solution each time, until the urine is clear and flowing freely.

13. Connect the new drainage bag.

Post procedure

Patient	Equipment/Environment	Nurse
• Ensure the patient is comfortable and is not experiencing bladder discomfort. • Encourage fluids and mobilisation if condition allows.	• Dispose of equipment and waste appropriately.	• Remove gloves and apron and wash hands. • Measure the input and output to calculate any urine output. • Document bladder washout and report any abnormalities.

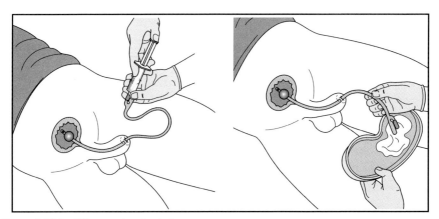

Figure 8.18 Instilling washout solution

Points for practice

1. Bladder washout or lavage using a syringe is undertaken mainly to remove blood clots following urological surgery. It should not be used to unblock long-term urethral catheters as the use of bladder syringes have been shown to cause damage; even the gentlest of force in instilling and withdrawing solution has been found to cause tissue trauma (Rew 2005).

2. A bladder-tip syringe differs from other syringes in that the tip is large and designed to fit the opening of a urinary catheter.

3. A broad selection of antibiotics and antiseptics has been used as bladder instillations with the aim of reducing infection and catheter blockage. However, there is evidence to suggest that there are no beneficial effects in preventing catheter-associated urinary-tract infections (Parkin & Keeley 2003). However, commercially prepared catheter maintenance solutions (CMS) are now being used in the management of long-term urethral catheters to dissolve encrustations, the most common cause of catheter blockage. These fluids are administered by gravity and under no circumstances should they be inserted into the bladder using a syringe (Rew 2005).

4. If no fluid is returned after instillation of the first 30 ml, instil a further 30 ml. If there is still no return, seek advice.

CATHETER REMOVAL

Preparation

Patient	Equipment/Environment	Nurse
• Explain the procedure, to gain consent and co-operation PFP1. • Ensure the patient's privacy and dignity are maintained throughout. • Position the patient in a supine position with knees and hips flexed and slightly apart.	• Clean trolley or tray. • A 20 ml syringe PFP2. • Large disposable absorbent pad. • Receiver. • Yellow waste bag for disposal of catheter and catheter bag. • Specimen pot and 20 ml syringe (for catheter specimen).	• Choose appropriate time for catheter removal PFP3. • Wash and dry hands thoroughly. • An apron and gloves should be worn.

Procedure

1. Take the equipment to the bedside.
2. Take a catheter specimen of urine (see page 201).
3. Place the disposable pad under the buttocks and the receiver between the patient's thighs.
4. Check the volume of water in the balloon (usually written on the catheter), attach the syringe to the balloon port on the catheter and withdraw the water to deflate the balloon PFP4.
5. Ask the patient to breathe in and out. As the patient exhales, gently but firmly withdraw the catheter into the receiver PFP4.

Post procedure

Patient	Equipment/Environment	Nurse
• Assist the patient into a comfortable position and ensure a lavatory or urinal/commode is nearby. • Advise the patient regarding the possibility of frequency, urgency, haematuria and dysuria PFP5. • Advise the patient to increase oral fluid intake (2–2.5 l in 24 hours). • Ask the patient to inform the nurse when urine has been passed.	• Dispose of equipment and waste appropriately.	• Remove gloves and apron and wash hands. • Record the amount of urine in the catheter drainage bag on the fluid balance chart. • Document the time of catheter removal and when the patient subsequently passes urine. • Label the catheter specimen and send it to the laboratory with the request form or refrigerate it as soon as possible.

Points for practice

1. The patient may be frightened of catheter removal and imagine it to be extremely painful.

2. The size of syringe required will depend on the amount of water in the catheter balloon; 10 ml is the recommended volume (Robinson 2004). This is written on the catheter itself.

3. Traditionally, catheters have been removed first thing in the morning. However, research has shown that midnight removal increases the length of time before passing urine, leading to a greater initial volume. This is said to aid a faster return to normal voiding and a reduction in anxiety (Kelleher 2002).

4. If problems are encountered when deflating the balloon or withdrawing the catheter, medical advice should be sought. Some research has indicated that following withdrawal of the water using a syringe, the catheter balloon membrane collapses, and deforms, resulting in creases and ridge formation. Therefore, it is essential that the catheter is withdrawn slowly and gently in order to reduce the trauma to the urethra caused by the creases and ridges in the balloon (Robinson 2003). Rotating the catheter as it is slowly withdrawn may also make removal easier.

5. The patient may well experience feelings of wanting to pass urine following removal of the catheter. Male patients should be discouraged from placing a urinal in position 'just in case', as this may encourage frequent small volumes to be passed or 'dribbling'. A frequency chart may be requested for the first 24 hours. Haematuria (blood in the urine) may be the result of trauma following catheter removal and dysuria (pain when passing urine) may be due to inflammation of the urethra.

STOMA CARE

Principles

- Stoma is a greek word meaning 'opening' or 'mouth' (Burch 2005a). The major types of surgically created stomas are: colostomy (opening into colon), ileostomy (opening into the ileum) or urostomy (e.g. ileal conduit – a stoma that drains urine). The most common type of stoma is a colostomy.

- In the immediate post-operative period, a baseline assessment of the stoma must be undertaken, which includes recording of the type of stoma, location, colour, size and length. In addition, while undertaking other post-operative observations, the nurse should observe the stoma. It should be pink or red in colour and the temperature of the stoma should be the same as the rest of the abdomen. This can be assessed by touching the stoma through a transparent appliance/bag (Burch 2005b).

- Day-to-day assessment should include: examination of the mucocutaneous junction (where the mucosa of the bowel joins the skin), assessment of the peristomal skin condition and the surface anatomy of the peristomal area (Burch 2005b). Output from the stoma should be noted and any concerns about the type or volume should be reported. It is important to clearly document observations and assessment.

- Regular care and inspection of a stoma is vital so that any deterioration in the stoma, such as mucocutaneous separation (stoma detaches from the edges of the surrounding skin and can leave a cavity), necrosis, prolapse, retraction, herniation or skin excoriation is reported promptly (Burch 2004). Delay exacerbates the problem and may cause pain and distress for the patient.

- Gloves and an apron should be worn when caring for a stoma. Additional protective clothing may be necessary if indicated by the patient's condition (see Chapter 9).

Stoma appliances

- There is an extensive range of stoma products available that are largely grouped into one-piece and two-piece appliances. One-piece appliances have the flange and pouch as one unit whilst they are separate in two-piece appliances. Hospitals tend to use transparent bags that facilitate observation of the stoma. These appliances usually come with a starter hole that allows the nurse to cut the flange to fit the size of the stoma; in the immediate post-operative period the stoma size changes as it settles down after surgery (Black 2000).

- Stoma appliances should be: leak proof, odour proof, unobtrusive, noiseless and disposable. In the first few days following surgery a flatus filter should not be used as it is important to observe when the bowel begins to work and produce flatus. Reassurance is important at this stage as the odour can cause the patient distress (Black 2000).

- When cutting the flange ensure it is cut according to the template so that it fits snugly around the stoma (Figure 8.19). If the aperture is too small, the edge of the aperture will cause friction on the delicate blood vessels of the stoma, causing bruising or bleeding (Burch 2004). If, on the other hand, the aperture is too big, the contents of the bowel will spill out of the stoma onto the surrounding skin, causing excoriation and soreness (Trainor et al 2003).

- When the bag is removed, it is important to do this gently so that the skin is not pulled (Trainor et al 2003). Use counter-pressure with your other hand.

- The skin and stoma should be cleaned whenever the bag is changed, to prevent skin soreness. A special stoma cream may be advocated if there are skin problems at the stoma site. Make sure the surrounding skin is dry before attaching a new bag.

- Ensure the bag is securely attached to the skin, thus preventing leakage and distress for the patient. Some stoma bags have a clip at the bottom to enable them to be emptied without removing the bag. Take care that the clip is securely fitted to prevent leakage.

- Many Trusts have a stoma nurse specialist for advice regarding care of the stoma.

CHANGING A STOMA BAG

Preparation

Patient	Equipment/Environment	Nurse
• Assist the patient to sit or lie in a comfortable position **PFP1**. • Ensure privacy and dignity are maintained throughout. • Place a protective pad next to the stoma site to protect clothing.	• Clean stoma bag and flange **PFP2**. • Scissors to cut the flange or aperture of the bag to the correct size. • Stoma template. • Tissues or gauze swabs. • Jug to dispose of the contents of the used bag. • Yellow clinical waste bag. • Soap and water for cleansing the skin. • Barrier cream If advised.	• Wash and dry hands thoroughly. • Put on apron and gloves. • Additional protective clothing may be necessary if indicated by the patient's condition (see Chapter 9).

Procedure

1. If the stoma bag is the type that can be emptied before removal, empty the contents of the stoma bag into the jug.
2. Gently peel the adhesive off the skin, using the other hand to apply counter-pressure.
3. Wipe the skin free of faeces and secretions using damp tissues or gauze **PFP3**.
4. Clean the skin and stoma using soap and water and dry well.
5. Check the condition of the stoma and the surrounding skin and apply barrier cream if appropriate.
6. Cut a hole to the correct size in the bag or flange using the stoma template as a guide.
7. Place the flange and/or the bag over the stoma so that the aperture fits snugly and is well attached **PFP4** (Figures 8.19 & 8.20).
8. If appropriate, attach the clip to the base of the bag **PFP5**.

Post procedure

Patient	Equipment/Environment	Nurse
• Offer the patient a hand wash if they have participated in the process. • Ensure the patient is comfortable.	• Dispose of excreta down the sluice. • Discard the soiled bag and other clinical waste appropriately. • Return unused equipment.	• Remove gloves and apron and wash hands. • Document the stoma bag change and report any abnormalities.

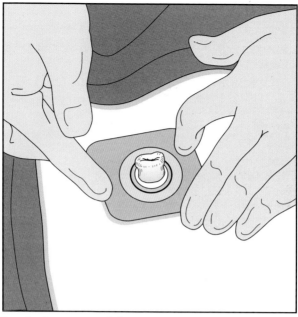

Figure 8.19 Fitting the flange around the stoma

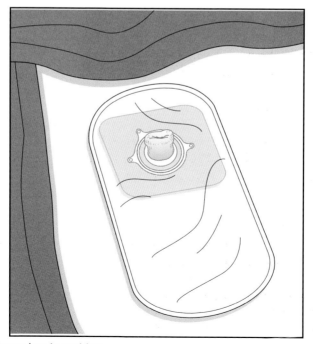

Figure 8.20 Stoma bag in position

Points for practice

1. Patients are usually taught to care for their own stomas and so should be encouraged to participate.

2. Many patients have a bag containing all the necessary equipment. Some stoma bags have a separate flange and bag; others are one-piece appliances (see page 233).

3. Cotton wool must not be used as it can leave wisps behind (Trainor et al 2003).

4. If a one-piece appliance is being used it should be applied from the bottom up. For a two-piece appliance, the flange should be placed directly over the stoma and the pouch attached (Trainor et al 2003).

5. If the bag is the type that can be emptied without removing it, there will be a special 'roll-up' clip at the bottom. Take care not to discard this when emptying the bag.

References and further reading

Black P. (2000) Practical stoma care. *Nursing Standard* **14**(41):47–55.

This article forms part of the Continuing Professional Development series and provides a comprehensive but practical overview of the issues facing patients with stomas.

Booth F, Lee L. (2005) A guide to selecting and using urinary sheaths. *Nursing Times Plus* **101**(47):43–46.

This article provides a good update on the issues to be considered when selecting urinary sheaths.

Burch J. (2004) The management and care of people with stoma complications. *British Journal of Nursing* **13**(6):307–318.

This article outlines the variety of complications that are associated with stomas. Actual and potential problems are discussed, ranging from the most common to the most rare. Possible solutions are offered as well as advice that may be offered by the nurse.

Burch J. (2005a) Exploring the conditions leading to stoma-forming surgery. *British Journal of Nursing* **14**(2):94–98.

This article explores the many reasons why a stoma may be formed. Although cancer is the most common, there are many other diseases of the gastrointestinal or urinary systems that may require temporary or permanent stoma formation. The nurse's role in caring for these patients is explored.

Burch J. (2005b) The pre- and postoperative nursing care for patients with a stoma. *British Journal of Nursing* **14**(6):310–318.

This article discusses the various issues that surround the nursing care of a patient with a stoma (colostomy, ileostomy or urostomy). The article outlines the anatomy, the stoma appliances and practical help in the pre- and postoperative care of an ostomate.

Department of Health. (2001) *The Essence of Care: continence and bladder and bowel care.* Department of Health, London.

Government guidelines based on patient-focused bench-marking to ensure high quality care.

Doherty W. (2006) Male urinary catheterisation. *Nursing Standard* **20**(35):57–63.

This article is part of the continuing professional development series. It examines the procedure of male catheterisation and its development as a role performed by trained nurses, regardless of gender. The reasons for urinary catheterisation, issues in relation to male sexuality and patient assessment and education are also discussed.

Head C. (2006) Insertion of a urinary catheter. *Nursing Older People* **18**(10):33–36.

This article focuses on the urinary catheter insertion in older people. The article explores the incidence of catheter use and associated complications. The correct procedure for catheter insertion is outlined.

Kelleher MB. (2002) Removal of urinary catheters midnight *vs* 0600 hours. *British Journal of Nursing* **11**(2):84–90.

This article reports on a prospective clinical trial to determine the impact midnight removal of urinary catheters would have on the patients' voiding patterns and subsequent discharge from hospital. The results indicate that midnight removal of urinary catheters leads to earlier resumption of normal voiding patterns, permits earlier discharge from hospital and appears to reduce patient anxiety.

Mangnall J, Watterson L. (2006) Principles of aseptic technique in urinary catheterisation. *Nursing Standard* **21**(8):49–56.

This article explains the principles of aseptic technique and its application to the procedure of urinary catheterisation.

Moppett S. (2000) Which way is up for a suppository? *Nursing Times* **96**(19):NT Plus:12–13.

This article discusses the rationale relating to the most effective way to insert a suppository (blunt end first) in order to aid retention.

O'Connor G. (2005) Teaching stoma-management skills: the importance of self-care. *British Journal of Nursing* **14**(6):320–324.

This article explores the importance of teaching stoma-management skills to patients beginning in the pre-operative period. The article outlines the importance of skills acquisition for the ostomate who has had to make major physical and psychological life adjustments.

Parkin J, Keeley FX. (2003) Indwelling catheter-associated urinary tract infections. *British Journal of Community Nursing* **8**(4):166–170.

This paper reviews the literature on the subject of catheter-associated urinary tract infections, with reference to the use and possible improvement of closed sterile catheter drainage systems.

Pomfret I. (2004) The use of anaesthetic gel for catheterization. *Nursing and Residential Care* **6**(8):383–386.

This article considers the use of lubricating anaesthetic gel in urinary catheterisation. While this is common practice for male catheterisation there is a view that it should also be the practice for female catheterisation.

Pomfret I. (2006) Urinary catheter care. *Nursing and Residential Care* **8**(10):446–448.

This article explores the use of indwelling urinary catheters to manage urinary incontinence when all else has failed. The advantages and disadvantages are explored as well as the methods, types of drainage systems and issues in respect of maintenance of the catheter.

Rew M. (2005) Caring for catheterized patients: urinary catheter maintenance. *British Journal of Nursing* **14**(2):87–92.

This article explores the evidence and opinions surrounding the ongoing problem of catheter blockage and how catheter life can be maintained. The article examines the role of pH testing, the role of the patient's general health, the use of catheter-maintenance solutions and techniques associated with instillations.

Rigby D, Gray K. (2006) Understanding urine testing. *Nursing Times* **101**(12):60–62.

This article looks at collection of urine specimens and urinalysis using reagent sticks. It also explains what abnormal findings might mean and the implications for practice.

Robinson J. (2003) Deflation of a Foley catheter balloon. *Nursing Standard* **17**(27):33–38.

This article reports a study undertaken to investigate the changes in urethral and suprapubic catheters following deflation and removal. The results of the study showed that manual syringe aspiration results in crease and ridge formation and an increase in catheter balloon diameter size on deflation and, therefore, has implications for the manner in which the catheter is removed.

Robinson J. (2004) Fundamental principles of indwelling urinary catheter selection. *British Journal of Community Nursing* **9**(7):281–284.

This article considers the importance of appropriate catheter selection. The article discusses the need for care in respect of catheter length, material, Charrière size and balloon infill volume as they are all likely to cause problems. Advice is offered on catheter selection and outlines what may occur if certain issues are dealt with incorrectly.

Robinson J. (2006a) Continence: sizing and fitting a penile sheath. *British Journal of Community Nursing* **11**(10):420–427.

This article discusses the importance of correct selection of a penile sheath. The article explains what is required before fitting a penile sheath, examines various sheaths and alternatives and outlines how to fit one correctly.

Robinson J. (2006b) Selecting a urinary catheter and drainage system. *British Journal of Nursing* **15**(19):1045–1050.

Selecting a catheter and drainage system can be confusing due to the vast array of catheters, materials used and drainage systems available from various companies. This article is written to help in the selection of a urinary catheter and the drainage system which is best suited to the patient.

Roodhourse A, Wellsted A. (2006) Safety in urine sampling: maintaining an infection-free environment. *British Journal of Nursing* **15**(16):870–872.

This article reports on a new needle-free port designed specifically to reduce the occupational health risk of needlestick injuries associated with urine sampling in patients with an indwelling urinary catheter.

Scholtes S. (2002) Management of clot retention following urological surgery. *Nursing Times* **98**(28):*NT Plus:*48–50.

This article addresses clot retention following urological surgery and includes discussion of continuous bladder irrigation and bladder washouts (lavage).

Selfe L. (2006) Disorders of the urinary system. In: Alexander MF, Fawcett JN, Runcimann PJ (eds). *Nursing practice hospital and home.* 3rd edn. Churchill Livingstone, Edinburgh.

This chapter provides a good overview of the anatomy and physiology urinary system and male reproductive system. It addresses common disorders of the urinary system (infections, renal disorders and disorders of the prostate) and has a good section on continuous bladder irrigation, choice of catheter size, etc., and post-op care following prostatectomy.

Skinner S. (2005) *Understanding clinical investigations: a quick reference manual.* 2nd edn. Baillière Tindall, Edinburgh.

This excellent book provides information about a wide range of investigations, why they are done, what the findings might indicate and the implications for nurses. It also provides a quick overview of the relevant physiology.

Trainor B, Thompson MJ, Boyd-Carson W, Boyd K. (2003) Clinical protocols for stoma care 2: changing an appliance. *Nursing Standard* **18**(13):41–42.

This article is part of the clinical protocols for stoma care and focuses on changing a stoma appliance. The technique for changing a stoma appliance is outlined with the aim of enabling nurses to teach patients how to manage their own stoma care.

Woodward S. (2005) Use of lubricant in female urethral catheterization. *British Journal of Nursing* **14**(19):1022–1023.

This article offers further support for the use of lubricant anaesthetic gel routinely for female patients who are undergoing urinary catheterisation. It is suggested that the procedure can cause physical trauma to the urethra and can be painful for the patient.

Wilson J. (2006) *Infection control in clinical practice.* 3rd edn. Baillière Tindall, Elsevier, Edinburgh.

A comprehensive text that explains basic microbiology, types of organisms and how they are spread. It then provides guidance on all aspects of infection control. Chapter 13 provides advice on cleaning, disinfection and sterilisation.

Notes

9

Prevention of cross-infection

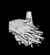

STANDARD PRECAUTIONS

Standard precautions are the standard infection control precautions that are essential in preventing cross-infection (*www.rcn.org.uk*). They include the precautions required when contact with body fluids is likely, previously called universal precautions. These precautions are:

- Cover all cuts, abrasions and lesions, especially those on the hands and forearms, with a waterproof dressing
- Maintain hand hygiene (hand washing or use of alcohol-based hand-rub) before and after each patient contact
- Maintain cleanliness of the environment
- Use disposable gloves and aprons when handling body fluids
- Use disposable aprons for direct patient care, bed making and aseptic techniques
- Dispose of waste safely
- Avoid overcrowding patients
- Avoid unnecessary transfer of patients between wards
- Isolate patients with a known or suspected infection.

METHICILLIN-RESISTANT *STAPHYLOCOCCUS AUREUS* (MRSA) AND *CLOSTRIDIUM DIFFICILE*

Methicillin-resistant *Staphylococcus aureus* (MRSA) and *Clostridium difficile* are both important causes of hospital-acquired infection (HAI). The most important route of transmission is on the hands of healthcare workers if not removed by hand washing. The use of alcohol-based hand-rub is effective against MRSA and so can be used instead of hand washing when the hands are socially clean. However, the spores of *C. difficile* can survive in the environment and are not killed by alcohol hand-rubs and so the hands must be washed with soap and water after contact with infected patients or their environment.

HAND WASHING

Preparation

Patient	Equipment/Environment	Nurse
• The hands should be washed before and after all patient contact **PFP1**.	• A sink with elbow- or foot-operated mixer taps is best.	• Remove any rings, jewellery and wrist watches **PFP3**.
	• Liquid soap or antiseptic detergent hand washing solution **PFP2**.	• Any cuts or abrasions on the hands should be covered by a waterproof, occlusive dressing.
	• Disposable paper hand towels.	• The fingernails should be short and no nail polish or artificial fingernails should be worn **PFP4**.
	• Foot-operated waste bins.	

Procedure

1. Adjust the taps so that the temperature is comfortable and the water flow is steady and does not result in splashing the surrounding area. Wet the hands.

2. Apply sufficient soap or antiseptic detergent solution to create a good lather.

3. Rub the hands briskly together, making sure that the thumbs, fingernails, fingertips, palms, backs of the hands and the wrists are thoroughly washed **PFP5**.

4. Scrubbing the skin is not recommended as it causes microabrasions. Only if the fingernails are visibly dirty should a nailbrush be used.

5. Continue to wash the hands for at least 10–15 seconds, then rinse thoroughly until all traces of soap/antiseptic detergent are removed **PFP6**.

6. Turn off the taps with your foot or elbow and allow the water to run off your hands by holding them with the fingers pointing upwards. If the taps are not elbow- or foot-operated, leave the water running until after drying your hands and then use a paper towel to turn off the taps.

7. Dry your hands using disposable paper towels, working from your fingertips towards the wrists. Thorough drying is essential to minimise the growth of micro-organisms and to prevent the hands becoming sore.

8. Discard the used paper towels according to local policy **PFP7**.

Points for practice

1. Alcohol hand-rub may be used instead of washing when the hands are socially clean. The alcohol must be applied to all areas (see page 244) and the hands then rubbed vigorously until dry. Alcohol effectively reduces microbial counts in clean hands, but it is ineffective if used on hands contaminated with

body fluids or excreta. Alcohol hand-rub alone is not effective against *Clostridium difficile* spores and should be used in addition to, not instead of, hand washing if *C. difficile* is present (*www.DH.gov*).

2. Bars of soap should never be used in clinical areas as they provide the ideal environment for growth of micro-organisms when left sitting on the sink in a pool of water. Liquid soap is usually sufficient for hand washing in most situations, but an antiseptic detergent hand washing solution containing chlorhexidine or iodine may be required before procedures such as urinary catheterisation. The local infection control policy will indicate when this is necessary.

3. Local policy may permit the wearing of a wedding ring. This should be a plain band and loose enough to allow washing and drying underneath it. Wrist watches must not be worn as they prevent effective washing of the wrist area.

4. Winslow and Jaconson (2000) reviewed several studies into the wearing of artificial nails and nail polish. They report that operating theatre personnel with artificial nails more often harboured gram-negative rods both before and after surgical scrubbing and artificial nails also had higher bacterial loads. Although the evidence about the effect of nail polish is unclear, they found that nurses with chipped nail polish had significantly more organisms than freshly polished or natural nails.

5. Several research studies have shown that hand washing techniques are not always effective. Areas of the hands that are commonly missed are the thumbs, fingernails, fingertips, palms, backs of the hands and the wrists (Figure 9.1) (Wilson 2006).

6. The hand washing technique should take at least 10–15 seconds (Cole 2007).

7. In some hospitals, hand towels are considered to be clinical waste and so should be discarded in the yellow clinical waste bag. In others they are deemed to be household waste and so should be discarded in the black non-clinical waste bag. Check your local policy.

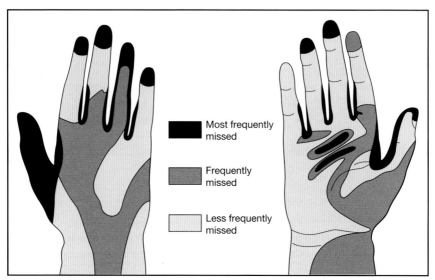

Figure 9.1 Areas often missed when the hands are washed

PERSONAL PROTECTIVE CLOTHING

Protective equipment is used to protect you and your patient from the risks of cross-infection. It includes aprons, gloves, goggles and visors, and in areas such as the operating theatre, may also involve the use of gown and hats (*www.rcn.org. uk*). Body fluids are a major source of micro-organisms associated with HAI and so protective clothing should be worn for any direct contact with body fluids. In order to decide whether additional protective clothing and eye protection is required you need to assess the risk of contact with body fluids and the risk of splashing (Wilson 2006) (see Figure 9.2).

Use of masks

Until fairly recently masks were used to prevent patients from micro-organisms from the respiratory tract of the staff caring for them and to protect staff caring for patients with infectious diseases. However, masks have been shown to be ineffective and are no longer routinely worn. Their use is only recommended in situations where there is a high risk of splashing of blood or other body fluids, for example in the operating theatre (Wilson 2006).

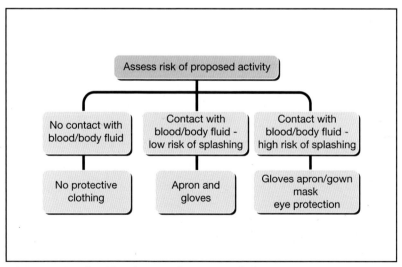

Figure 9.2 Assessing the risk: selection of protective clothing

USE OF APRONS

Preparation

Patient	Equipment/Environment	Nurse
• Aprons should be worn in all situations where there is direct patient contact or contact with body fluids, bed linen, excreta, clinical waste, etc., or with items that have been in contact with infectious diseases, such as clothes, books, etc.	• Plastic aprons may be available in a variety of colours. In some hospitals, a system exists whereby different coloured aprons are used for specific purposes, e.g. for serving meals or performing dressings.	• The apron should be put on after the hands have been washed.

Procedure

1. Wash and dry your hands thoroughly.
2. Pull the apron over your head; avoid touching your hair and clothing if possible.
3. Tie the apron loosely at the back to avoid it becoming gathered at the waist, so that water splashes will run off easily.
4. If gloves are required (see page 247), put them on after the apron and remove them before the apron is removed at the end of the procedure **PFP1**.
5. To remove the apron, pull at the top and the sides to break the neckband and waist-ties, and fold the apron in on itself to prevent the spread of micro-organisms **PFP2**. Do not allow your hands to touch your uniform.
6. Discard the used apron into the yellow clinical waste bag.
7. Wash and dry your hands thoroughly (see page 242).

Points for practice

1. Your gloves are likely to be more heavily contaminated than your apron. Removing your gloves before the apron reduces the risk of contamination of your clothing when breaking the neckband and waist-ties to remove the apron.
2. Folding the apron carefully as it is removed reduces the risk of shaking organisms into the air and your hands only touch the 'clean' side of the apron.

USE OF GLOVES (NON-STERILE)

Preparation

Patient	Equipment/Environment	Nurse
• Gloves should be worn whenever patient care involves dealing with blood or other body fluids.	• Seamless, single-use latex gloves are recommended. These fit either hand and are available in three sizes: large, medium and small **PFP1**.	• The use of gloves does not reduce the need for hand washing. The hands should be washed before and after gloves have been worn **PFP2**.
• Gloves may also be required when there is any contact with a patient who has an infection, such as hepatitis, methicillin-resistant *Staphylococcus aureus* (MRSA) or *Clostridium difficile*.		
• Check whether the patient has a latex allergy **PFP1**.		

Procedure

1. It is important to choose the correct size of glove; otherwise dexterity will be severely impaired.
2. If the gloves are required for a 'clean' procedure, such as blood glucose monitoring, they should be taken from those stored in a clean area where they are protected from dust.
3. When removing gloves, do not touch your wrists or hands with the dirty gloves. Using a gloved hand, pinch up the glove of the other hand at the wrist and pull it off turning it inside out. With the non-gloved hand, slip your fingers into the wrist of the other glove and pull it off, again turning it inside out (Figure 9.3).
4. Used gloves must be discarded in the yellow clinical waste bag.
5. Wash and dry the hands thoroughly **PFP3**.

Points for practice

1. It is important to check whether the patient has a latex allergy (Hampton 2002). Latex-free gloves should be available in all clinical areas but may need to be specially ordered. If you have a known latex allergy it is wise to inform the clinical area in advance when possible.

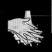

2. The hands must be washed before and after gloves are worn because the hands sweat within the gloves, creating a warm, moist environment, which encourages micro-organisms to multiply (Allen 2005). Also, gloves may not completely protect the hands – they have been shown to develop tiny punctures that go undetected but allow micro-organisms to pass through (Hampton 2002). For information on the use of sterile gloves see page 261.

3. If an apron is worn, this should be removed after the gloves, but before the hands are washed (see page 247).

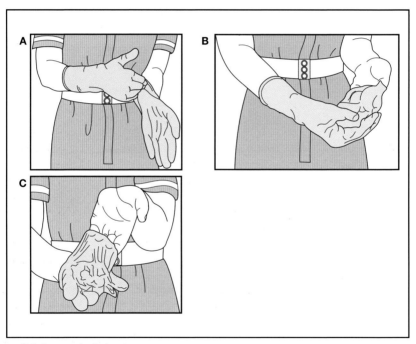

Figure 9.3 Removal of gloves

DISPOSAL OF WASTE AND CARE OF EQUIPMENT

Clinical waste

Any waste generated in healthcare settings that has been in contact with blood or other body fluids is classed as clinical waste and must be incinerated. This includes soiled dressings, swabs, catheters, urine drainage bags, sputum pots, incontinence pads, etc. Used aprons and gloves are also likely to be contaminated by blood or other body fluids and so these should also be classed as clinical waste. All clinical waste must be placed in **yellow plastic bags** for incineration (DH 2006).

Non-clinical waste

Waste generated in hospital that poses no risk to others is classed as non-clinical waste and may be disposed of in the same way as normal household waste. This includes waste such as paper hand towels, newspapers, dead flowers, food packaging, etc. Non-clinical waste should be placed in **black plastic bags** for disposal (DH 2006).

Needles and other sharps

Many healthcare procedures involve the use of needles or other devices capable of puncturing the skin, such as scalpels, lancets, etc., which are collectively referred to as 'sharps'. An injury from a needle or other device contaminated with blood or other body fluids poses a high risk to healthcare workers and so special care must be taken when using and disposing of sharps (May & Brewer 2001). All sharps must be discarded into special yellow sharps bins, which are rigid, puncture resistant and leak proof (Figure 9.4). They have a special opening that is designed to allow sharps to be dropped easily into the container, but will not allow items to spill out should the container topple over. Sharps bins must not be filled more than three-quarters full, and once closed, they cannot be reopened.

Used needles must never be resheathed and should not be separated from the syringe except when used for venepuncture (see page 66). If removal of the needle from the syringe is necessary, a sharps bin with a needle-removing facility on the top should be used so that the needle is not handled (Figure 9.4). The safe disposal of needles and other sharps is always the responsibility of the person who used them; they should never be left for anyone else to clear away. Where possible, the sharps bin should be taken to the place where the sharps will be used, as this allows immediate disposal after use. If this is not possible, a rigid tray or receiver should be used to contain the sharps until they can be safely tipped, without further handling, into the sharps bin. Items **must never be forced** into an already full container, as this may result in injury.

Linen

Used linen

This refers to all bed linen, clothing, towels, etc., that has been used by patients, but is not soiled. A plastic apron should be worn when making beds and handling used

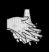

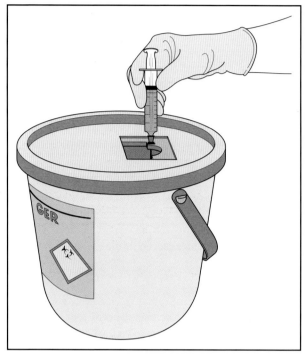

Figure 9.4 Safe disposal of sharps

linen to prevent contact with your uniform, and gloves will be necessary if the patient has an infection, such as MRSA or *C. difficile*, even when the linen is not soiled. Used linen should be placed in a polythene or fabric linen-bag. These bags must not be overfilled and should be securely fastened to prevent spillage of the contents. Check clothing, such as pyjamas, to ensure that objects, such as spectacles or hearing aids, are not in the pocket.

Soiled or fouled linen

This refers to linen contaminated with blood or other body fluids or excreta. To prevent leakage, this linen should be placed in a plastic bag (often red but the colour may vary according to local policy), which should be sealed and then placed in a linen-bag as described above. Personnel wearing protective clothing and gloves will deal with soiled or fouled linen in the laundry.

Infected linen

This refers to linen from patients with infectious conditions, such as salmonella, hepatitis, pulmonary tuberculosis or MRSA. This linen must be placed in a plastic bag with a water-soluble seam and then placed in a special fabric linen-bag, which is often red or has red markings on it. In the laundry, the infected linen is not handled by anyone, but put straight into a high-temperature (95°C) washing machine in its plastic bag. The water-soluble seam will dissolve during the wash, allowing the linen to be laundered (Wilson 2006).

Non-disposable equipment

Although the majority of clinical equipment is now disposable, some items are designed to be reused, and this requires sterilisation in the sterile supplies department of the hospital. Such equipment (e.g. surgical instruments, vaginal speculae, etc.) should not be washed after use, but placed immediately in a clear plastic bag and returned to the appropriate department for decontamination. There is usually a system whereby all such equipment is placed in a particular bin or bag (the colour of this will vary according to local policy), to await collection for cleaning and sterilisation. Items of equipment that are identified as single-use equipment must never be decontaminated and then reused for another patient (Wilson 2006). Item such as nebulisers (see page 310) can be reused several times by the same patient before being discarded.

General equipment

Equipment such as washbowls, commodes, beds and mattresses must be cleaned thoroughly between patients to avoid cross-infection (Wilson 2006). These should be cleaned with alcohol wipes or detergent and hot water, and dried thoroughly (refer to local policy). The use of detergent is essential for effective cleaning as it breaks up grease and dirt and improves the ability of water to remove it (Wilson 2006). All equipment should be stored clean and dry between uses. Many hospital wards provide patients with individual washbowls, which are kept in the bedside locker. However, others keep a number of bowls for communal use in the sluice. Abrasive materials should not be used to clean plastic washbowls as this roughens the surface, making it easy for micro-organisms to become trapped. Once washed, bowls should be placed upside down in a pyramid to allow the air to circulate freely and they dry thoroughly (Wilson 2006). The Royal College of Nursing (RCN) has useful guidelines for the decontamination of equipment and a table to help you determine the appropriate decontamination method according to whether equipment is a high, medium or low risk (*www.rcn.org.uk/infectioncontrol*).

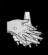
TAKING A SWAB

Preparation

Patient	Equipment/Environment	Nurse
• Explain the procedure, to gain consent and co-operation.	• Sterile swab.	• Wash and dry hands thoroughly.
• Ensure comfort and privacy are maintained.	• Plastic specimen bag.	• Put on apron and gloves.
	• Laboratory request form.	

Procedure

1. Ask/assist the patient to adopt a position that allows access to the appropriate site **PFP1**.

2. Open the packaging at the handle end and remove the swab, taking care not to contaminate the absorbent tip **PFP2**.

3. Twist the end of the swab between your finger and thumb to 'roll' the swab so that all areas of the absorbent tip come into contact with the designated area. Avoid touching the surrounding skin **PFP3**.

4. Open the transport tube and carefully insert the swab. The 'handle' of the swab becomes the stopper or cap of the tube (Figure 9.5).

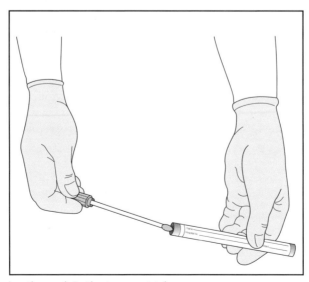

Figure 9.5 Placing the swab in the transport tube

Post procedure

Patient	Equipment/Environment	Nurse
• Ensure the patient is comfortable.	• Label the specimen container **PFP4** and place it in a plastic specimen bag with the laboratory request form and dispatch to the laboratory or refrigerate as soon as possible. • Dispose of clinical waste appropriately.	• Remove gloves and apron and wash hands. • Document that the swab has been taken.

Points for practice

1. For MRSA screening, swabs are usually taken from the nose, throat, perineum and any wounds. A specimen of urine will also be required if the patient is catheterised (see page 198). Refer to local policy for the sites to be swabbed.

2. The swab may come packed inside its transport tube or it may be packed separately.

3. If the swab is being taken when performing an aseptic dressing technique, this should be done before cleaning/irrigating the wound with antiseptic solution. However, some authors suggest that removal of exudate prior to swabbing allows access to the organisms actually causing the wound infection, which are different from those in the exudate at the surface of the wound (Starr & Macleod 2003). If there is no exudate, the tip of the swab may be moistened with transport medium supplied in the tube or 0.9% sodium chloride.

4. The patient's details should include: surname; first name; date of birth; hospital number; ward; date and where the swab was taken from (e.g. axilla).

References and further reading

Allen G. (2005) Hand hygiene, an essential process in the OR. *AORN* **82**(4):561–562.

Demonstrates that wearing gloves creates a moist, warm, nutrient-rich environment in which bacteria can grow and multiply, and stresses the need for hand washing before and after wearing gloves.

Department of Health (2006) *Technical Memorandum 07-01: Safe Management of Healthcare Waste*. Available from the Department of Health website (see below)

A comprehensive document that covers all aspects of waste management in healthcare, within hospitals and in community settings.

Cole M. (2007) Should nurses take a pragmatic approach to hand hygiene? *Nursing Times* **103**(3):32–33.

An interesting article, which argues that recommended practice standards in relation to hand hygiene can be unrealistic and lead to non-compliance. By developing a more pragmatic approach this may lead to better compliance and an overall improvement in standards.

Gould D. (2002) Hand decontamination. *Nursing Times* **98**(46):48–49.

Gould D. (2002) Preventing cross infection. *Nursing Times* **98**(46):50–51.

These two articles outline the hand washing technique and discuss when soap is sufficient and when antiseptic solutions should be used. They also discuss use of gloves, care of the nails and the wearing of rings and wrist watches.

Girou E, Loyeau S, Legrand P, Oppein F, Brun-Buisson C. (2002) Efficacy of hand rubbing with alcohol based solution versus standard hand washing with antiseptic soap: a randomised clinical trial. *BMJ* **325**:362–364.

An interesting study conducted in three intensive care units in France, which found that the reduction in bacterial contamination of the hands was significantly higher when alcohol-based solution was used rather than hand washing.

Hampton S. (2002) The appropriate use of gloves to reduce allergies and infection. *British Journal of Nursing* **11**:1120–1124.

This article discusses appropriate and inappropriate use of gloves and the issues surrounding the use of latex and this may impact on the nurse, patient and the environment.

Infection Control Nurses' Association (2002) *Protective clothing: principles and guidelines*.

Practical evidence-based guidelines regarding the appropriate use of protective clothing as part of infection prevention and control.

May D, Brewer S. (2001) Sharps injury: prevention and management. *Nursing Standard* **15**(32):45–53.

A continuing professional development article to help you review the risks associated with needlestick injury and blood-borne viruses and develop safe systems of working. Also discusses what to do if a sharps injury occurs.

O'Connor H. (2000) Decontaminating beds and mattresses. *Nursing Times* **96**(46):NTPlus:2–5.

This article defines the terms decontamination, cleaning, disinfection and sterilisation and provides a practical guide to the decontamination of beds and mattresses.

Pratt R, Pellowe C, Loveday H, Robinson N, Smith GW and the *epic* guideline development team. (2001) The EPIC project: developing national evidence-based guidelines for preventing healthcare associated infections. *Journal of Hospital Infection* **47**(Supplement): S3–S4. Also available at *www.doh.gov.uk/HAI*.

Evidence-based guidelines for preventing infections in hospitals and HAIs associated with urethral catheters and central venous catheters.

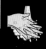

Raybould LM. (2001) Disposable non-sterile gloves: a policy for appropriate use. *British Journal of Nursing* **10**(17):1135–1141.

Reports an audit of glove use in which it was found that gloves were sometimes being used inappropriately. Provides a good overview of when they should be worn and a nice diagram, based on work by the ICNA, to show which type of gloves should be worn for which activity.

Roberts M. (2001) Reservoir bugs: sources of hospital-acquired infection. *Nursing Times* **97**(46):*NTPlus*:54–55.

A useful summary of what is meant by HAI (hospital/healthcare-acquired infection) and ways that clinical equipment can act as a reservoir for infectious organisms.

Starr S, MacLeod T. (2003) Wound swabbing technique. *Nursing Times* **99**(5):57–59.

This article reviews the evidence to support whether to cleanse a wound prior to taking a wound swab and the technique that should be used. It also reports a study into nurses' knowledge of the rationale underpinning swab technique.

Wilson J. (2006) *Infection control in clinical practice*. 3rd edn. Baillière Tindall, Elsevier, Edinburgh.

A comprehensive text that explains basic microbiology, types of organisms and how they are spread. It then provides guidance on infection control practices, disposal of waste, decontamination of equipment and advice about all aspects of infection control.

Winslow E, Jacobson A. (2000) Can a fashion statement harm the patient? *American Journal of Nursing* **100**(9):63–65.

This article reviews several studies into the effects of artificial and polished nails on hand-hygiene practices. They conclude that artificial nails could contain more bacteria than natural nails and so place patients at increased risk of infection. The evidence regarding the use of nail polish is less clear, but they recommend that if polish is worn it should be freshly applied and clear so that the nails can be inspected for cleanliness.

Websites

www.rcn.org.uk

The Royal College of Nursing website provides a lot of guidance about all aspects of infection control, hand washing technique, standard (universal) precautions and MRSA. Many of the resources are freely available to non-members.

www.icna.org

The website of the Infection Control Nurses' Association and has free downloads of audit tools, core competencies, etc.

www.doh.gov

The website of the UK Department of Health has a good overview of MRSA and *Clostridium difficile* and how they are spread. Also, latest figures on infection rates in hospitals, etc., and good practice guidelines.

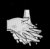
 Notes

10

Wound assessment

ASEPTIC DRESSING TECHNIQUE

Preparation

Patient	Equipment/Environment	Nurse
• Explain the procedure, to gain consent and co-operation.	• Dressing trolley or other suitable surface.	• Consult the care plan to determine the type of dressing required, frequency of change, etc.
• Assess the wound dressing PFP1.	• Dressing pack, syringe (for irrigating the wound), cleansing solution and new dressing according to the care plan/local policy PFP2.	• Make sure hair is tied back securely.
• Check patient comfort, e.g. position, convenience, need for toilet, etc.		• Wash and dry hands thoroughly.
• Administer analgesics as appropriate and allow time to take effect.	• Alcohol hand-rub or hand washing facilities.	• An apron should be worn. Additional protective clothing may be necessary if indicated by the patient's condition (see Chapter 9).
	• Draw screens around the bed and ensure adequate light. Clear the bed area, close windows, turn off fans, etc.	
	• Adjust bedclothes to permit easy access to the wound but maintain warmth and dignity PFP3.	

Procedure

1. Clean the trolley or other appropriate surface according to local policy PFP4.

2. Gather the equipment, check the sterility and expiry date of all equipment and solutions. Place these on the bottom of the trolley or somewhere convenient.

3. If scissors are needed to cut non-sterile tape, wash your own scissors, dry them thoroughly and then clean them with an alcohol-impregnated swab. If sterile scissors are needed (e.g. to cut a sterile dressing), these may be included in the dressing pack or packed separately.

4. Take the trolley to the bed area PFP5. Adjust the bed to a safe working height to avoid stooping.

5. Remove the dressing pack from its outer packaging; place it on the clean trolley/surface.

6. Remove the yellow waste bag and place it to one side. This may not be possible until after step 7.

7. Using your fingertips and touching the edges of the paper only, open the pack and lay it flat to create a sterile field (Figure 10.1).

8. Touching only the wrist part of the gloves (or edge of glove pack) move them to the edge of the sterile field (see Figure 10.1).

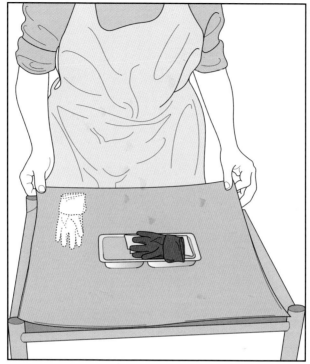

Figure 10.1 Opening the dressing pack

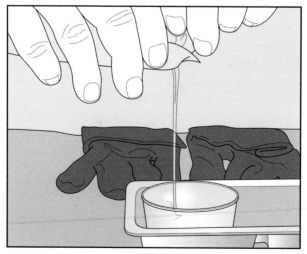

Figure 10.2 Pouring the cleansing solution

9. Taking care not to contaminate the sterile field, carefully pour the cleansing solution into the tray (Figure 10.2). Open the dressing, syringe, etc., onto the sterile field. If non-sterile tape is to be used, cut/tear it now and attach it to the trolley in a convenient place for use later.

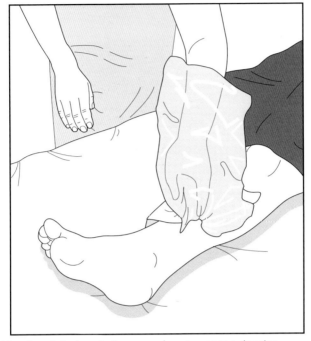

Figure 10.3 Using the clinical waste bag as a glove to remove dressing

10. Adjust any remaining bedclothes to expose the wound then loosen the existing dressing, but do not remove it PFP6.

11. Wash your hands or use alcohol hand-rub. Ensure your hands are completely dry before proceeding.

12. Open the yellow waste bag and put your hand inside so that the bag acts as a glove. Use this to remove the soiled dressing (Figure 10.3).

13. Inspect the dressing to determine the type and amount of exudate.

14. Turn the bag inside out so that the dressing is contained within it, and using the self-adhesive strip, attach the bag to the side of the trolley or other convenient place close to the wound PFP7.

15. Taking care not to touch the outside of the gloves, put on the sterile gloves (Figure 10.4).

16. Use a gauze swab dipped in cleansing solution to clean *around* the wound to remove blood, etc. PFP8.

17. If the wound itself needs cleaning, use a syringe primed with solution in one hand and a gauze swab on the skin below the wound in the other (Figure 10.5). Making sure that neither the syringe nor gauze come into contact with the wound, allow the solution to flow into the wound, collecting the solution in the gauze swab held below the wound.

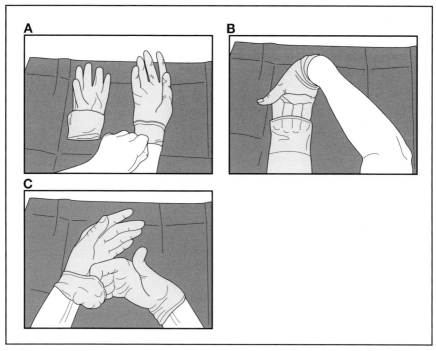

Figure 10.4 Putting on sterile gloves

18. Use fresh gauze swabs to dry *around* the wound (not the wound itself), using each swab once only and swabbing away from the wound.

19. Apply the new dressing. Remove gloves and discard into waste bag.

Post procedure

Patient	Equipment/Environment	Nurse
• When the dressing is secure, replace the bedclothes and assist the patient as necessary into a comfortable position. • Readjust the bed to a safe height.	• Wrap all used disposable items in the sterile field and place in the waste bag. This should then be tied and placed in the clinical waste. • Place any sharps, e.g. stitch cutters, in a sharps bin.	• Remove apron and wash hands. Return any unused items to the stock cupboard. • It is not necessary to clean the trolley again unless it has become wet or contaminated with body fluids (Wilson 2006). • Document the care given and the condition of the wound. Report any changes or abnormalities.

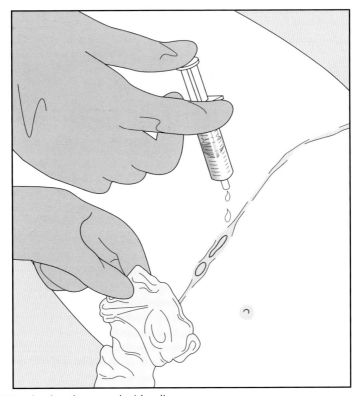

Figure 10.5 Irrigating the wound with saline

Points for practice

1. Examine the care plan and the current dressing to determine what type is being used and whether it has been adequate, e.g. whether more padding to absorb exudate is needed.

2. The type of dressing pack will vary according to availability, individual preference and the type of wound.

3. Do not leave the patient unattended on a raised bed. Leave the screens only partly drawn until you return if there are concerns about patient safety.

4. The trolley or surface used must be cleaned thoroughly before use. Local policies may vary, but hot soapy (detergent) water is recommended and the surface must then be dried thoroughly to discourage the growth of micro-organisms (Wilson 2006). If alcohol wipes are indicated in the policy, those designed for hard surfaces (not skin wipes) must be used and allowed to dry thoroughly.

5. In some hospitals, dressings are performed in a clean treatment room rather than at the bedside, to reduce the risk of cross-infection.

6. Leave the existing dressing in place to minimise wound exposure to airborne organisms and minimise wound cooling as this affects wound healing (Wilson 2006).

7. The waste bag should be positioned so that used swabs can be disposed of without passing over the sterile field.

8. Gauze should not be used to clean inside the wound as this has been shown to damage the delicate granulating tissue of a healing wound. In some hospitals the solution is warmed to prevent cooling and vasoconstriction at the wound site.

9. A syringe (usually 10 ml unless the wound is very large) should be used to irrigate gently any wound that needs cleaning. There is a lack of agreement regarding the recommended pressure to use when irrigating the wound (Dearden et al 2001).

REMOVAL OF SKIN CLOSURES: SUTURES/STAPLES

Preparation

Patient	Equipment/Environment	Nurse
• Explain the procedure, to gain consent and co-operation.	• Dressing pack containing sterile gloves.	• Consult the care plan to determine when the sutures/staples are due for removal, the dressing type, etc.
• Check patient comfort, e.g. position, convenience, need for toilet, etc.	• Sterile scissors/stitch cutter and forceps or staple remover as appropriate.	
• Administer analgesics if appropriate and allow time to take effect PFP1.	• Alcohol hand-rub or hand washing facilities.	• Make sure hair is tied back securely.
	• Draw screens around the bed and ensure adequate light. Clear bed area, close windows, turn off fan, etc.	• Wash and dry hands thoroughly. An apron should be worn.
	• Adjust the bedclothes to permit easy access to the wound but maintain warmth and dignity PFP2.	• Additional protective clothing may be necessary if indicated by the patient's condition (see Chapter 9).

Procedure

1. Follow the procedure for the aseptic dressing technique to step 9 (see page 258).
2. Taking care to maintain sterility, open the stitch cutter and forceps or staple remover onto the sterile field (Figure 10.6).
3. Adjust any remaining bedclothes to expose the wound then loosen the existing dressing but do not remove it.
4. Wash your hands or use alcohol hand-rub. Make sure that your hands are completely dry before proceeding.
5. Open the sterile waste bag and put your hand inside so that the bag acts as a glove (see Figure 10.3). Use this to remove and inspect the old dressing.
6. Turn the bag inside out so that the dressing is contained within it, and using the adhesive strip, attach the bag to the side of the trolley or other convenient place close to the wound PFP3.
7. Taking care not to touch the outside of the gloves, put on the sterile gloves (see Figure 10.4).
8. Inspect the wound for signs of healing. If the wound looks inflamed or there is any exudate (pus) present, advice should be sought from an experienced nurse. It may be necessary to remove just one or two sutures/staples to allow the pus to drain PFP4.
9. Do not clean the wound before removing the sutures/staples, as cleansing solution may seep into the holes made by the sutures/staples when removed.

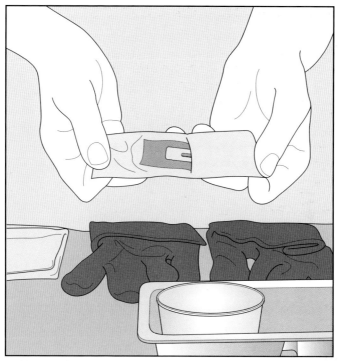

Figure 10.6 Adding stitch cutter to the sterile field

10. If the wound is longer than 15 cm, remove alternate sutures/staples and check that the wound is fully healed before removing the rest **PFP5**:

- **Individual sutures** – use the forceps to lift up the knot of the suture. In your other hand, hold the scissors or stitch cutter flat against the skin and slide it under the suture to cut it (Figure 10.7A). The place where you cut it is important; in order to prevent infection the part of the suture that has been lying on the skin must not be drawn underneath the skin and so the place where it is cut is important.

- **Staples** – a special instrument is used to remove staples (Figure 10.7B). This should be placed under the centre of the staple and squeezed hard. This bends the staple so that it comes out of the skin easily and does not have to be 'hooked' out. The staple can be steadied, if necessary, by holding it with forceps.

- **Continuous suture** – this means the incision is held together with one thread, which passes under and over the incision about every centimetre. There is a knot at each end. Use the forceps to lift the knot at one end and cut the first 'suture' at the end furthest from the knot (Figure 10.8a). Lift the knot to remove the loose end from under the skin and cut close to the skin (Figure 10.8b). Slide the forceps under the next stitch (Figure 10.8c), raise it to remove the underlying thread and cut it close to the skin. Repeat this process with all the others, making sure that the part that has been on the skin is not pulled underneath the skin. Never cut both ends of a suture or you will be unable to remove the hidden part underneath the skin.

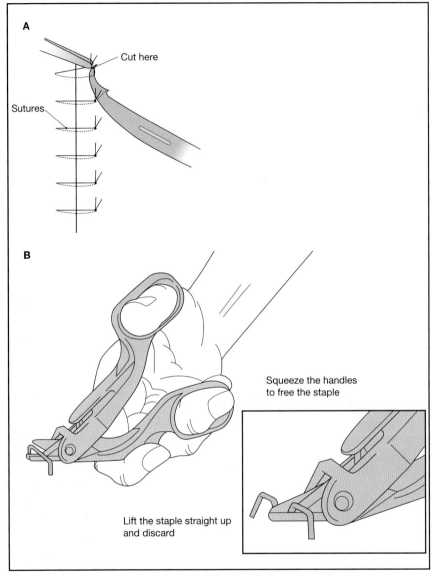

Figure 10.7 (A) Individual suture removal, (B) removal of staples

- **Subcutaneous suture** – this is a continuous suture but it is not visible above the skin. There is usually a bead at each end. Cut the thread holding one bead and gently pull the other until the whole thread is removed from under the skin.
11. Use a gauze swab soaked in cleansing solution to clean and then dry around the wound if necessary (not the wound itself).

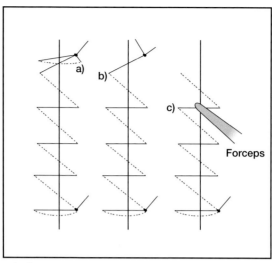

Figure 10.8 Removal of continuous suture

12. If there are any small areas where the skin edges are not completely healed together, skin-closure strips may be applied PFP6.

13. If appropriate, apply the new dressing. Remove gloves and discard into clinical waste bag.

Post procedure

Patient	Equipment/Environment	Nurse
• Replace the bedclothes and assist the patient as necessary into a comfortable position.	• Wrap all used disposable items in the sterile field and place in the waste bag, which should then be tied and placed in the clinical waste.	• Remove apron and wash hands. Return any unused items to the stock cupboard.
• Readjust the bed to a safe height.		• It is not necessary to clean the trolley again unless it has become wet or contaminated with body fluids (Wilson 2006).
	• Place any sharps, e.g. stitch cutters, in a sharps bin.	• Document the care given and the condition of the wound. Report any changes or abnormalities.

Points for practice

1. The removal of sutures or staples should not be painful, although the patient may anticipate pain or discomfort. Explanation and careful positioning may alleviate this.

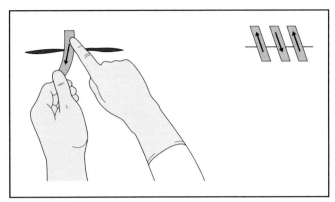

Figure 10.9 Applying skin-closure strips

2. Do not leave the patient unattended on a raised bed. Leave the screens only partly drawn until you return if there are concerns about patient safety.

3. The waste bag should be positioned so that used swabs can be disposed of without passing over the sterile field.

4. If the wound is longer than 15 cm or if the incision is in a place where there may be a strain on the skin and underlying tissues, it is better to remove alternate sutures/staples, starting with the second one along. This allows you to check that the wound does not begin to gape at any point before the rest are removed. If the wound begins to gape, the remaining sutures/staples may be left until the following day and reassessed. In some instances the number of sutures/staples removed needs to be documented. With continuous sutures (see step 10), if the wound begins to gape do not remove any more. Make sure it is clear where the free end is and the rest can be left in place.

5. When removing sutures only make one cut until you can determine where the loose end is and it is visible. The part of the suture that has been lying on the skin must not be pulled under the skin during removal as this will introduce micro-organisms into the skin.

6. Skin-closure strips are used to pull the edges of the wound together to promote healing. Attach the strip to the skin on one side of the wound and making sure that the skin edges are aligned without creating excessive tension, lay it over the wound and attach it to the skin on the other side. The next and any subsequent strips should be attached first to alternate sides of the wound (Figure 10.9). This is designed to apply even pressure to the wound edges.

WOUND DRAINAGE

Principles

Open system

- This refers to a hollow tube or corrugated piece of rubber or plastic that is situated in the wound to promote drainage into the dressing (Figure 10.10). If there is a large amount of drainage, the end of the drain may be inserted into a stoma bag (see page 233). This is designed to keep the wound area free from drainage and thus reduce the risk of infection and to prevent damage to the skin.

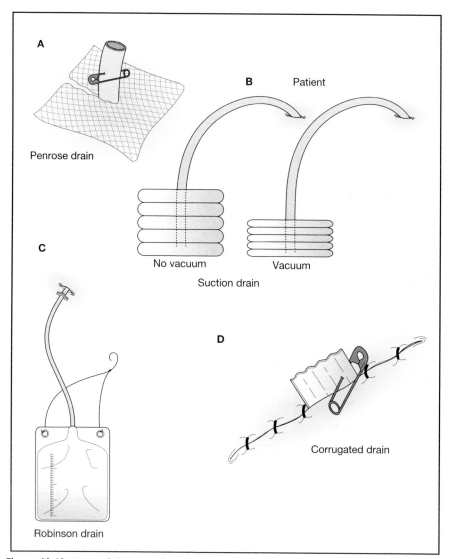

Figure 10.10 Types of drain available

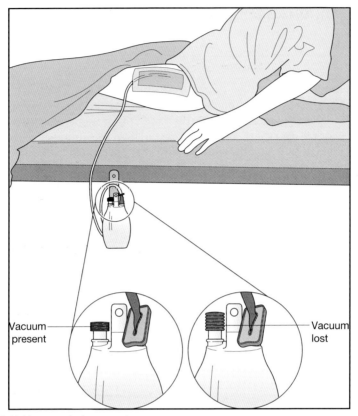

Figure 10.11 Vacuum drainage system

Closed system

- This refers to a system whereby the drain is attached to tubing and a bag for the collection of drainage. This means that the system is 'closed' and thus the risk of infection is greatly reduced. Many closed systems incorporate a vacuum to encourage drainage (Figure 10.11).

- The bag or bottle should be supported by attachment to the bed or patient's clothing to prevent pulling and accidental dislodgement of the drain.

- Asepsis must be maintained when changing the bag or bottle (see page 271).

CHANGING A VACUUM DRAINAGE BOTTLE

Preparation

Patient	Equipment/Environment	Nurse
• Explain the procedure, to gain consent and co-operation.	• New vacuum drainage bottle (check that a vacuum is present) `PFP1`. • Yellow clinical waste bag.	• Wash and dry hands thoroughly. • Put on apron and clean gloves. • If there is a danger of splashing, goggles should be worn `PFP2`.

Procedure

1. Detach the drainage bottle from the bed, taking care not to let the bottle slip or the drainage tube may be pulled out.
2. With the clamps that are provided as part of the system, clamp off both the drainage tube (above the connection to the bottle) and the bottle.

Bottle system

3. Carefully remove the drainage tube from the 'old' bottle, taking care not to touch the last 2–3 cm to keep it sterile.
4. Note the volume of drainage, then discard the bottle with its contents into the clinical waste bag `PFP3`.
5. Push the tubing firmly into the new bottle and release the vacuum clamp. Release the clamp on the drainage tubing.
6. Secure the bottle to the bed or patient's clothing to prevent pulling.

Small concertina system

3. If drainage is no longer required, remove the drainage tubing and insert the stopper. Discard into the clinical waste system. If it is necessary to empty the drainage and replace the vacuum container, detach the container, empty into a jug taking care to avoid splashing.
4. Squeeze the container flat, push the tubing firmly back into container and release the clamp on the drainage tubing.
5. Secure the container to the bed or patient's clothing to prevent pulling.
7. Remove gloves, discard into clinical waste bag and close securely.

Post procedure

Patient	Equipment/Environment	Nurse
• Ensure the patient is comfortable and the drain is not pulling.	• Dispose of equipment and clinical waste appropriately.	• Remove apron and wash hands. • Document the amount and type of drainage.

Points for practice

1. The presence of a vacuum is usually indicated by the small concertina of plastic folds at the top of the bottle; when the vacuum is no longer present, the concertina effect is lost (Figure 10.11). If only a small amount of drainage is expected, a small concertina container may be used. This is squeezed flat to create a vacuum and then the stopper is replaced to maintain the vacuum.

2. If there is a risk of splashing during the bottle change, goggles should be worn. However, nurses who wear spectacles do not need to wear goggles (see Chapter 9).

3. The used bottle, once clamped, should be discarded into the yellow clinical waste bag. It should not be emptied because of the risk of splashing and contact with blood.

REMOVAL OF A DRAIN

Preparation

Patient	Equipment/Environment	Nurse
• Explain the procedure, to gain consent and co-operation.	As for the aseptic dressing technique (see page 258) plus:	• Wash and dry hands thoroughly.
• Prepare the patient as described on page 258.	• Sterile stitch cutter or sterile scissors.	• Put on apron.
	• Sterile forceps.	• Additional protective clothing may be necessary if indicated by the patient's condition (see Chapter 9).
	• Sterile dressing towel.	

Procedure

1. Prepare the patient, bed area and equipment as described for the aseptic dressing technique (see page 258).

2. Note the amount of drainage. If the drain has a vacuum bottle attached, clamp the tubing with the clamp provided to prevent suction during removal of the drain **PFP1**.

3. Put on sterile gloves and clean the site, if necessary, so that the knot of the suture holding the drain in place is visible and accessible **PFP2**. Place the sterile towel under the tubing.

4. Lift up the knot of the suture with the sterile forceps, and using the stitch cutter, cut the suture close to the skin, and remove the suture (see page 265).

5. Fold a gauze swab several times to create an absorbent pad and hold this over the site.

6. Warning the patient of a pulling sensation, gently remove the drain onto the sterile towel. Use counter-pressure on the skin with the other hand if resistance is felt **PFP3**.

7. Maintain pressure over the site until bleeding/drainage is minimal. Cover the site with a sterile dressing.

8. Detach the bottle from the bed/clothing. Wrap the bottle and the tubing in the sterile towel and discard into the clinical waste bag.

9. Remove gloves and discard with dressing pack into the clinical waste bag and close securely.

Post procedure

Patient	Equipment/Environment	Nurse
• Ensure the patient is comfortable.	• Dispose of all sharps and other clinical waste appropriately. • Scissors, if not disposable, should be returned to the sterile supplies department for decontamination.	• Remove apron and wash hands. • Document the time and date of removal, and the amount and type of drainage.

Points for practice

1. Clamping the tubing prevents suction during removal, which may be painful for the patient.
2. If the drain site appears inflamed or purulent, a swab for culture and sensitivity should be taken (see page 248).
3. Check that the entire drain has been removed. If the drain cannot easily be removed, leave it in position and report it to the nurse in charge.

References and further reading

Baxter H. (2003) Management of surgical wounds. *Nursing Times* **99**(13):66, 68.

  A useful article that examines the intrinsic and extrinsic factors that affect wound healing, such as skin preparation and shaving, and complications such as dehiscence.

Collier M. (2003) The elements of wound assessment. *Nursing Times* **99**(13):48–49.

  This article provides a good overview of the holistic assessment of wounds and includes classification, assessment of the surrounding skin, using photographic records and documentation.

Dealey C. (2005) *The care of wounds: a guide for nurses.* Blackwell Publishing, Oxford.

  A comprehensive book that covers the history of wound care, physiology of wound healing, types of dressings and all types of wounds including pressure ulcers and even skin care for patients undergoing radiation.

Dearden C, Donnell J, Donnelly J, Dunlop M. (2001) Traumatic wounds: cleansing and dressing. *Nursing Times* **97**(28):50, 52.

  Although the focus is on traumatic wounds most of this article is equally applicable to all wounds. It addresses wound cleansing, irrigation and different types of wound closure.

Morris D, Ward K. (2004) Perioperative nursing. In: Brooker C, Nicol M (eds) *Nursing Adults; the practice of caring.* Mosby, Elsevier, Edinburgh.

  Chapter 29 addresses all aspects of peri-operative nursing including wound care and management of wound drains.

Hoban V. (2005) Wound care; what every nurse should know. *Nursing Times* **101**(12):20–22.

  An interesting article that argues that wound care is every nurse's responsibility, not just the responsibility of the specialist tissue-viability nurses. It discusses evidence-based practice, type of dressing and their uses and the early warning signs that something is going wrong.

Johnstone C, Farley A, Hendry C. (2005) The physiological basis of wound healing. *Nursing Standard* **19**(43):59–65.

  This is part of the Continuing Professional Development series and provides a good overview of the A & P of the skin and the wound healing process.

Patel S, Beldon P. (2003) Examining the literature on using tap water in wound cleansing. *Nursing Times* **99**(43):22–24.

  Reviews the literature on use of tap water in chronic wounds and concludes that there is insufficient robust evidence to either support or refute the use of tap water, but its use in chronic wounds such as leg ulcers it is probably appropriate.

Notes

11

Patient hygiene

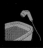

ASSISTING WITH A BATH OR SHOWER

Preparation

Patient	Equipment/Environment	Nurse
• Discuss the patient's preference for a bath or a shower PFP1. • Discuss/assess how much the patient is able to do for themselves and how much assistance may be required. • Ascertain whether the patient wishes to use the toilet before taking them to the bathroom. • Explain the procedure, to gain consent and co-operation.	• Soap/shower gel or antiseptic cleansing agent, according to local policy PFP2. • Flannel/sponge and towels. • Brush and/or comb. • Toothbrush, toothpaste and denture pot if appropriate. • Shampoo (if required). • Clean clothing. • Toiletries, make-up, etc., according to individual preference. • Shower stool or plastic chair. • Hoist and/or other aids to mobility as required.	• Put on plastic apron. • Additional protective clothing may be necessary if indicated by the patient's condition (see Chapter 9).

Procedure

1. Check that the bathroom is available and that the bath/shower is clean.

2. Run the bath water.

3. Help the patient to collect together clothes and toiletries.

4. Assist the patient to the bathroom and make sure that access by others is restricted, to ensure privacy.

5. For bathing: use your elbow to check that the bath water is the appropriate temperature (40°C) for the patient or a bath thermometer may be used PFP3.

6. Assist the patient with undressing, maintaining dignity by covering them with a towel.

7. Observe the condition of the patient's skin, especially at the pressure points such as heels and sacrum (see page 344). Note any signs of inflammation, bruising, discoloration or rash. Note the integrity of the skin and its hydration, whether dry, clammy or sweaty, etc.

8. For bathing: assist the patient to get into the bath. A mechanical hoist is likely to be required for immobile patients.

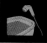

For showering: assist the patient to sit on the shower stool or chair and adjust the water flow to the correct temperature.

9. Assist the patient to wash. Encourage patients to do as much as they can themselves `PFP4`.

10. If required, assist the patient to wash their hair, using the flannel as an eye-guard to avoid getting shampoo in the eyes.

11. Assist the patient to get out of the bath or shower, using a mechanical hoist if required. Cover the patient with a towel as soon as possible, to provide warmth and maintain dignity.

12. Help the patient to: dry themselves; apply toiletries as requested; dress in chosen clothing; brush or comb their hair; clean their teeth or dentures as appropriate.

13. Assist the patient to return to bed, chair or day room, using a mechanical hoist if required.

Post procedure

Patient	Equipment/Environment	Nurse
• Ensure the patient is comfortable.	• Return/replace towels, toiletries, clothing, etc., as appropriate. • Clean the bath or shower.	• Record the procedure in the nursing documentation, noting how much assistance the patient required, the state of the patient's skin and pressure points, and the patient's general condition. • Report any changes or deterioration.

Points for practice

1. If a shower is not available some patients may prefer to use running water while sitting in an empty bath. This is may be a culturally determined practice related to the requirement to perform ablutions prior to prayer.

2. Some Trusts require patients to use antiseptic cleansing solution rather than soap, as prophylaxis against methicillin-resistant *Staphylococcus aureus* (MRSA).

3. The hands can usually tolerate higher temperatures than the rest of the body. The elbow is more sensitive and will minimise the risk of the water being too hot. The safest option is to use a bath thermometer.

4. If leaving patients to wash themselves make sure they have access to a call bell for assistance.

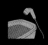
BED BATH

Preparation

Patient	Equipment/Environment	Nurse

Patient

- Discuss the procedure, to gain co-operation and consent.
- Ascertain if the patient wishes to use a bedpan/urinal or commode prior to their bed bath.
- The patient requiring a bed bath will be quite dependent and possibly confused or unconscious.
- Ensure privacy, warmth and dignity.

Equipment/Environment

- Close windows and switch off fans.
- Soap or antiseptic cleansing agent PFP1.
- Flannel and disposable cloths.
- Two towels.
- Toiletries, make-up, etc., according to individual preference.
- Brush and/or comb.
- Toothbrush and toothpaste, tumbler of water and bowl/receiver.
- Bowl of water (hand hot).
- Clean night clothes.
- Trolley or suitable work surface.
- Linen bag and bags for fouled or infected linen if required.
- Clean bed linen.
- Clinical waste bag.

Nurse

- An understanding of the patient's individual needs and preferences.
- A plastic apron should be worn.
- Gloves are not necessary to wash the body unless required by the patient's condition, e.g. MRSA or *Clostridium difficile* or if the patient has been incontinent PFP2.
- Two nurses may be required for this procedure PFP3.

Procedure

1. Assist the patient into a comfortable position. Clear space at bedside for bowl of water and toiletries.

2. Assist the patient to remove any night clothes, ensuring the patient is covered with a sheet or blanket to maintain warmth and dignity.

3. Assist the patient to wash the face, ears and neck. If soap is used, rinse well and dry thoroughly.

4. Wash, rinse and dry the body in a logical order, exposing only the part of the body to be washed. The suggested order is arms, chest, abdomen, genital area, legs, feet and then back PFP4; however, this should be discussed with the patient to ascertain any preferences. Change the water as it cools or becomes dirty. If two nurses are present, one should wash and rinse while the other dries the body and applies toiletries as requested, e.g. talc, deodorant or body cream. This reduces the amount of time the body is exposed.

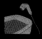

5. As the patient is washed, observe the condition of the skin. Note any signs of inflammation, bruising, discoloration or rash. Note the integrity of the skin and its hydration, e.g. whether dry, clammy or sweaty, etc.

6. Put on gloves and assist the patient to wash, rinse and dry the genital area using a disposable cloth. Remember to wash from the front of the perineal area to the back. In males, ensure that the foreskin is repositioned after washing and dry underneath it. If a urinary catheter is in place, wash carefully around the urethral meatus and catheter tubing, moving away from the meatus, and dry carefully (see page 216). Change the water after washing the genital area.

7. Assist the patient to put on night clothes.

8. Remove any soiled bed linen and remake the bed. This is likely to require a second nurse.

9. Assist the patient to clean teeth or dentures (see page 285). If the patient is going to sit out of bed after the bed bath, it is often easier to clean the teeth when sitting in a chair.

10. Assist the patient to brush or comb hair and to clean and file nails if necessary (see page 293).

Post procedure

Patient	Equipment/Environment	Nurse
• Ensure the patient is comfortable and has required belongings within reach.	• Wash and dry the bowl (see page 251). • Rinse the flannel under running water to remove all soap and allow it to dry. • Discard disposable cloths into the clinical waste. • Return the linen bag to its collection point.	• Remove apron and wash hands. • Record the procedure in the nursing documentation, noting how much the patient could do without assistance and the condition of the skin, eyes, mouth, etc.

Points for practice

1. Some Trusts require patients to use an antiseptic cleansing solution instead of soap as part of their infection control policy. Patients may prefer not to use soap on their face and, if they have any skin condition, may use an emulsifying ointment in the water instead of soap.

2. Gloves should be worn when washing the genital area as there is a risk of being contaminated with body fluids. Discard gloves prior to continuing to wash other parts of the body.

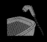

3. A bed bath can be carried out by one nurse, but for severely weak or unconscious patients two nurses are required.

4. The back is left until last so that it can be washed and the clean sheet inserted at the same time, to prevent unnecessary movement for the patient. One nurse can often manage until this point, but will need assistance to roll the patient and make the bed with clean linen.

ORAL ASSESSMENT

Preparation

Patient	Equipment/Environment	Nurse
• Explain the procedure, to gain consent and co-operation. • Ask the patient to sit upright if their condition allows.	• Pen torch or other suitable light source. • Tongue depressor.	• Wash and dry hands thoroughly. • Gloves and an apron should be worn. • Additional protective clothing may be necessary if indicated by the patient's condition (see Chapter 9).

Procedure

1. Observe the patient's lips, noting whether they are normal or dry and whether there is any evidence of ulcers, sores, cracks or bleeding.

2. Ascertain whether the patient has any dentures. Note their fit and then ask the patient to remove them. Note the condition of the dentures: whether they are clean, stained, warped or cracked.

3. Place the dentures in water, as they will become warped if left dry for long periods.

4. Put on gloves and using the torch, inspect the patient's teeth, noting any decay, white patches (oral thrush), plaque or debris (food) that may be trapped between the cheek and the gum **PFP1**. Identify any worn or loose teeth.

5. Using the tongue depressor and torch, inspect the inside of the mouth, paying attention to the gums, tongue and mucous membranes **PFP2**. Observe whether they are moist, pink and healthy looking or whether there are any blistered, ulcerated or cracked areas. Note any inflammation, swelling or bleeding of the gums and mucous membranes. Note the presence of any halitosis.

6. While inspecting the mouth, note the consistency and amount of any saliva that is present **PFP3**.

7. Ascertain whether the patient has any difficulty with speech, chewing or swallowing.

8. Discuss the patient's usual oral hygiene measures and assess whether assistance will be required with oral hygiene.

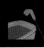

Post procedure

Patient	Equipment/Environment	Nurse

Patient

- Offer the patient water to rinse the mouth.
- Explain any further interventions that might be necessary.
- Ensure the patient is comfortable.

Equipment/Environment

- Clear away equipment.
- Discard gloves into the clinical waste.

Nurse

- Wash and dry hands thoroughly.
- Liaise with medical staff if any medication or referrals are required.
- Document the oral assessment in the nursing records.

Points for practice

1. Following cerebrovascular accident (stroke) patients often need assistance to check that food is not trapped as they may be unable to detect it.
2. If the patient is unconscious, two nurses may be required – one to carry out the assessment and one to support the patient's jaw during inspection.
3. In older patients xerostomia (reduced salivary flow) is particularly common (Coleman 2002).

MOUTH CARE FOR A DEPENDENT PATIENT

Preparation

Patient

- Explain the procedure, to gain consent and co-operation.
- Ensure privacy.
- Help the patient into a comfortable sitting position. If the patient is unconscious, position them on their side.

Equipment/Environment

- Towel and tissues.
- Toothbrush (preferably soft with a small head; may be battery operated).
- Toothpaste/denture cleaning paste.
- Container for dentures if required.
- Beaker of water and bowl or receiver.
- Mouthwash solution (e.g. glycothymoline) if required **PFP1**.
- Cleansing agent (e.g. weak sodium bicarbonate) if required **PFP2**.
- Foam sticks if required.
- Lip lubricant if required.
- Suction equipment if required.
- Clinical waste bag.

Nurse

- Wash and dry hands thoroughly.
- Put on gloves and apron.
- Additional protective clothing may be necessary if indicated by the patient's condition (see Chapter 9).

Procedure

1. Cover the patient's chest with a towel. If the patient is unconscious, cover the bed/pillow with a waterproof cover and a towel.

2. If applicable, remove the patient's dentures and place them in clean water.

3. Using a toothbrush and small amount of toothpaste, clean the teeth, gums and tongue, taking care not to cause any trauma to the mouth. Small side-to-side or circular strokes are the most effective **PFP3**. Remember to clean both the inner and outer aspects of the teeth **PFP4**.

4. If the mouth is encrusted with tenacious mucus or trapped food, a weak solution of sodium bicarbonate may be used **PFP2** – dip foam sticks into a freshly made solution and gently wipe these around the mouth **PFP5**.

5. Following cleaning, the mouth should be rinsed with water to remove any debris or remaining toothpaste, which can have a drying effect on the oral mucosa. The patient should be encouraged to rinse vigorously and then spit the fluid into a bowl. If the patient is unconscious, the mouth should be rinsed by using foam sticks dipped in water. Gentle suction may be used to remove fluid or excess secretions (see page 319).

6. If the patient has dentures, these should be cleaned with a toothbrush and denture-cleaning paste and rinsed thoroughly before giving them back to the patient. Ordinary toothpaste should not be used as this is too abrasive. Do not dry the dentures as this makes them difficult to insert PFP6.

7. If the lips are dry, a thin layer of petroleum jelly or lip balm may be applied.

Post procedure

Patient	Equipment/Environment	Nurse
• Ensure the patient is comfortable.	• Rinse the toothbrush and replace the toothbrush and toothpaste in the patient's locker.	• Remove gloves and apron and wash hands.
• Inspect the mouth (see page 283).	• Discard, or if required frequently, cover any unused cleaning solution PFP7.	• Document any abnormalities or improvements in the patient's oral condition in the nursing records.
	• Discard used equipment into the clinical waste.	

Points for practice

1. Some patients may prefer to rinse their mouth with a mouthwash solution after their teeth and mouth have been cleaned. This is very refreshing, but the effect is only short-lived and so mouthwash needs to be offered frequently.

2. If sodium bicarbonate solution is required, a weak solution should be prepared by mixing a very small amount (equivalent to 1 teaspoon in 500 ml) in a tumbler of water. If the solution is too strong it may damage the oral mucosa.

3. Some electric/battery operated toothbrushes have a variety of speeds. Set the brush at the lowest speed to minimise risk of traumatic injury.

4. If patients have oral thrush (*Candida albicans*), their dentures should be soaked in a chlorhexidine solution for at least 10 minutes to minimise the risk of re-infection.

5. A toothbrush is always preferable. Foam sticks are not effective in removing plaque from the surface of teeth but they are useful for rinsing or refreshing the mouth.

6. Unconscious patients should not wear their dentures, as these may obstruct the airway. The dentures should be cleaned and stored in water in a labelled denture pot.

7. Any solutions prepared for mouth care must be kept covered between uses and should be discarded and replaced every 24 hours.

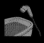

FACIAL SHAVE

Preparation

Patient

- Ascertain the patient's preferences for shaving and incorporate this into the hygiene routine accordingly.
- If possible, the patient should be sitting up.

Equipment/Environment

- Bowl of hot water.
- Flannel/disposable cloth and towel.
- Shaving cream or soap.
- Razor **PFP1**.
- Aftershave/cologne according to individual preference.

Nurse

- Wash and dry hands thoroughly.
- Put on apron.
- Additional protective clothing may be necessary if indicated by the patient's condition (see Chapter 9).

Procedure

1. Drape a towel across the patient's chest.
2. Ask/assist the patient to wash their face. Inspect the face for any raised areas, such as moles or sores.
3. Apply the shaving cream or soap to the face, creating a good lather.
4. Using short strokes of the razor in the direction of the hair growth, shave the face starting with the cheeks and moving down towards the neck **PFP2**. Avoid any raised area such as moles or blemishes.
5. The nurse's free hand should be used to pull the skin taut (Figure 11.1).
6. Rinse the razor after each stroke.

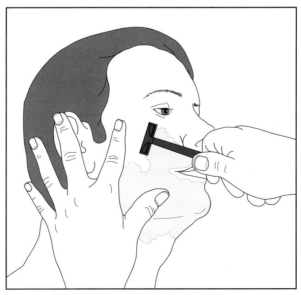

Figure 11.1 Holding the skin taut when shaving

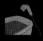

*7. When the entire face and neck have been shaved, rinse the face in clean water and pat dry with a towel.

8. Apply aftershave or cologne if desired.

Post procedure

Patient	Equipment/Environment	Nurse
• Ensure the patient is comfortable.	• Wash and dry the bowl and replace it in the appropriate storage area (see page 251).	• Remove apron and wash hands.
	• Rinse the flannel or discard the disposable cloth.	• Document the procedure, noting how much the patient could do unassisted.
	• Discard the razor or dulled razor blades into a sharps bin.	
	• Replace any personal equipment in the patient's locker.	

Points for practice

1. Many patients will have their own electric razor and so will not require a wet shave. Communal electric razors should not be used, because of the risk of cross-infection. Some depilatory creams are available for the face, but these must be patch tested 24 hours prior to use in case of allergic reaction.

2. Patients can often help by making facial movements that tighten the skin being shaved, e.g. filling out cheeks with the tongue.

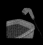

WASHING HAIR IN BED

Preparation

Patient	Equipment/Environment	Nurse
• Explain the procedure, to gain consent and co-operation.	• Plastic sheeting and absorbent pad or towel to protect the bed.	• A second nurse may be needed, to support the patient's head and neck.
• Ascertain the patient's preferences regarding hair care.	• Shampoo and conditioner if used.	• An apron should be worn.
• Ensure warmth and privacy.	• Comb and/or brush.	• Additional protective clothing may be necessary if indicated by the patient's condition (see Chapter 9).
	• Flannel/disposable cloth and towels	
	• Two large plastic bowls (one full of hand-hot water, the other empty) PFP1.	
	• Clean jug.	
	• Hairdryer if available.	

Procedure

1. Remove the head of the bed.
2. Place the plastic sheeting and the absorbent pad or towel over the pillows, and place the empty bowl on a chair at the top of the bed.
3. Ask/assist the patient to lie on their back at the very top of the bed, with pillows supporting the shoulders and the head positioned over the bowl. Cover the shoulders with a towel (Figure 11.2).

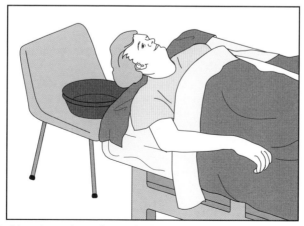

Figure 11.2 Washing the patient's hair in bed

4. Observe the condition of the hair and scalp **PFP2**. Wet the patient's hair by taking warm water from the bowl into the jug and pouring it over the hair, allowing the water to run into the bowl on the chair.

5. Gently massage shampoo into the hair.

6. Rinse the hair with clean water, ensuring that the patient protects their eyes with the flannel or disposable cloth to avoid shampoo getting in. Repeat the process if the patient would like two applications of shampoo and/or conditioner.

7. If conditioner is used, comb it through the hair and leave for 2–3 minutes before rinsing.

8. After the final rinse, wrap the patient's hair in a towel and remove the bowl of water.

9. Assist the patient into a sitting position (if their condition allows) and towel dry the hair.

10. Brush or comb the hair into the desired style, using a hairdryer if one is available **PFP3**.

Post procedure

Patient	Equipment/Environment	Nurse
• Ensure the patient is comfortable and in a warm environment until the hair is dry.	• Replace the head of the bed and arrange the pillows. • Dispose of equipment and used towels appropriately. • Wash and dry bowls and jug, and replace them in the storage area (see page 251).	• Remove apron and wash hands. • Record the procedure in the nursing documentation.

Points for practice

1. Some hospitals provide an inflatable hair-washing device that collects the water and so only one bowl is necessary.

2. Before washing the hair, the nurse should assess the condition of the scalp, noting any inflammation, dryness or redness. The condition of the hair should also be noted.

3. Some patients may like products applied to their hair after washing to prevent dryness and help with styling.

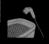

EYE CARE

Preparation

Patient	Equipment/Environment	Nurse
• Explain the procedure, to gain consent and co-operation PFP1. • Assist the patient into a comfortable position, with the head tilted backwards.	• Sterile eye-care pack containing gallipot, gauze swabs and a dressing towel PFP2. • Extra gauze swabs if required. • Sterile 0.9% sodium chloride (normal saline) solution. • Clinical waste bag.	• Wash and dry hands thoroughly. • Apron and gloves should be worn. • Additional protective clothing may be necessary if indicated by the patient's condition (see Chapter 9).

Procedure

1. Open the eye-care pack and arrange all equipment on a suitable work surface.

2. Pour the saline solution into the gallipot.

3. Ask the patient to close their eyes, and explain which eye is to be cleaned first. Always clean an infected eye last PFP3.

4. Lightly moisten a gauze swab with saline, and swab the lower lid from the nose outwards, ensuring that the swab does not rise above the margin of the lid as this could cause corneal damage.

5. Using a new swab each time, repeat step 5 until any discharge or encrustation has been removed.

6. Repeat steps 5 and 6 with the upper lid.

7. Dry the lids by gently wiping with a dry swab.

8. Repeat steps 5–8 with the other eye PFP3.

Post procedure

Patient	Equipment/Environment	Nurse
• Ensure the patient is comfortable.	• Discard equipment into the clinical waste PFP4.	• Remove gloves and apron and wash hands. • Record the procedure in the nursing documentation, noting the condition of the eyes.

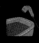

Points for practice

1. Eye care may be required prior to the administration of eye drops or ointment (see page 163).

2. If an eye care pack is not available individually packed sterile equipment can be assembled.

3. If both eyes are infected, two separate eye-care packs should be used and the hands washed and new gloves put on before cleaning the second eye.

4. Because of the risk of infection, eye-care packs should not be kept for repeated use. A new pack should be used each time.

CARING FOR FINGERNAILS AND TOENAILS

Preparation

Patient

- Explain the procedure, to gain consent and co-operation **PFP1**.
- Ascertain usual nail-care habits.
- Carry out this procedure following a bath if possible, as soaking will soften the nails.

Equipment/Environment

- Bowl of warm water.
- Nail file or emery board.
- Orange stick.
- Hand cream or lotion according to patient preference.
- Towel.

Nurse

- Wash and dry hands thoroughly.
- Put on plastic apron.
- Knowledge of local policy regarding nail care **PFP1**.

Procedure

Fingernails

1. Inspect the hands, fingers and nails, noting any signs of dryness and the condition of the nails and cuticles.
2. If patient has not recently had a bath soak the hands in a bowl of warm water for 15 minutes, re-warming the water as necessary.
3. Clean under the fingernails with an orange stick or nail file while the fingers are soaking.
4. Remove the fingers from the bowl and dry them thoroughly.
5. File the fingernails until they are level with the top of the finger. The nails can then be smoothed to the shape of the finger.
6. Push the cuticles back gently with an orange stick.
7. Apply hand cream or lotion as appropriate.

Toenails

1. Inspect the feet and toenails, noting any dryness, inflammation or cracking. Also note any calluses or ulcerated areas and the colour and temperature of the feet to assess adequacy of circulation.
2. If the patient has not recently had a bath, soak the feet in a bowl of warm water for 15 minutes, re-warming the water as necessary.
3. Clean and file the toenails as for fingernails, but do not file the corners as this may encourage ingrowing nails. If nails require cutting, the patient should be referred to the chiropodist.

Post procedure

Patient	Equipment/Environment	Nurse
• Ensure the patient is comfortable.	• Wash and dry the bowl and replace it in the appropriate storage area (see Care of general equipment, page 251).	• Remove apron and wash hands.
	• Replace any personal equipment in the patient's locker.	• Document the procedure in the nursing records and report any abnormalities, e.g. areas of ulceration or poor peripheral circulation (Popoola & Jenkins 2005).
	• Discard waste into the clinical waste.	

Point for practice

1. Most Trust policies state that patients must be referred to chiropodists and that nurses should not cut nails. This is especially important in patients with diabetes and peripheral arterial disease who may have peripheral neuropathy and, therefore, be unaware of any trauma to the toes.

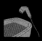
LAST OFFICES

Preparation

Patient

- Death will have been confirmed **PFP1**.
- Relatives will have been informed and given the opportunity to see the deceased and may wish to participate in the last offices.
- Attention must be paid to the beliefs and wishes of deceased patients and their relatives. Religious requirements should be observed. Advice from religious personnel may be required **PFP2**.
- Screen the bed securely as soon as death occurs.

Equipment/Environment

- Prepare the bed area to ensure sufficient space is available.
- Equipment for bed bath (see page 280).
- Cotton wool, gauze or padding as required.
- Clean sheet and counterpane.
- Tape for securing the sheet.
- Two name bands.
- Two labels from the 'deceased patients book' **PFP3**.
- Property book.
- Shroud.
- Small cotton bandage.
- Kidney dish (to express bladder).
- Linen bag and clinical waste bag.
- Cadaver bag (if required).

Nurse

- Last offices require two nurses working together quietly.
- Be familiar with hospital policy regarding last offices.
- An apron should be worn and gloves should be available.

Procedure

1. Take the equipment to the bedside and secure the screens, to prevent accidental opening.

2. Wash the front of the patient. The second nurse may be shaving the patient whilst the first nurse washes them. Leave/replace dentures if they fit.

3. Remove any tubes, catheters and infusions unless otherwise indicated, e.g. post-mortem (autopsy) requirements **PFP4**.

4. If leakage is apparent from wounds or orifices, use packing or padding, according to local policy **PFP5**. It may be necessary to express urine from the bladder into the receiver.

5. With the second nurse as a witness, remove all jewellery from the body unless advised otherwise, e.g. Sikhs – leave bracelet (kara). If jewellery is left, this should be covered with adhesive tape or tied in position to prevent loss.

6. Place the shroud on the patient, with the fastening at the back. Roll the patient onto their side to wash back and fasten shroud.

7. Place a clean sheet under the patient, leaving enough sheet to fold over the head and feet **PFP6**. Use the bandage to tie the feet together.

8. Place one label on the chest attached to the shroud with adhesive tape.

9. Place one nameband on the wrist and the other on the ankle or according to local policy.

10. Before wrapping the patient in the sheet, check if the relatives wish to view the body **PFP7**.

11. Wrap the body in the sheet and secure with tape.

12. Place the other label on the chest.

13. If there is a risk of infection, the body may be placed in a cadaver bag. The bag is labelled 'Danger of Infection' plus the name of the infection.

13. Complete the property form. Both nurses must document and sign for any valuables. Any valuables left on the body should also be noted on the death form.

Post procedure

Patient	Equipment/Environment	Nurse
• Pack the patient's belongings.	• Clear away equipment and dispose of clinical waste safely.	• Remove gloves and apron and wash hands.
• Store property according to local policy, e.g. in the bereavement office.	• Leave the area tidy, ready for cleaning/disinfecting.	• Complete the care plan and other documentation according to local policy.
• Contact porters or mortuary technicians to remove the body.	• Flowers, if present, may be left on the bedside locker.	
	• Ensure that the remaining patients' bed areas are screened when the body is removed, and a calm and quiet approach is adopted.	

Points for practice

1. After death, the body is usually left for an hour before last offices are commenced, during which time a doctor or senior nurse will have certified the death. A pillow may be used to support the jaw, to prevent the mouth falling open, and the eyes closed with wet gauze swabs if necessary. The limbs should be straightened if necessary.

2. Religious/cultural preferences must be ascertained prior to last offices, e.g. who can touch the body, non-removal of religious objects or jewellery, etc. (McGee 2002).

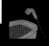

3. The labels used to identify the body are found in the 'deceased patients' or 'death notice' book and must be completed before being torn out, to ensure that all copies are completed at the same time. In some Trusts, the labels are provided with other items (e.g. shroud) in a 'last offices' pack.

4. The medical team will advise if a post-mortem is required.

5. It is important to prevent leakage from the body, as this is unpleasant and potentially dangerous for porters and mortuary technicians.
Refer to local policy regarding packing the body to prevent leakage.
This should not be performed if a post-mortem examination (autopsy) is required.

6. When rolling the patient to put in the clean sheet, a deep sigh may be heard. This is due to air being forced out of the lungs.

7. If the patient is to be seen by the family after last offices, a coloured counterpane makes the bed look less clinical.

References and further reading

Bailey R, Ledikwe J, Smiciklas-Wright H. (2005) The oral health of older adults: an interdisciplinary mandate. *Journal of Gerontological Nursing* **31**(7):11–17.
A useful article exploring the consequences of poor oral health care. Recommendations for practice are made.

Birrell J, Thomas D, Jones C. (2006) Promoting privacy and dignity for older patients in hospital. *Nursing Standard* **20**(8):41–46.
This article explores several ways of promoting dignity in older people and is especially relevant in relation to hygiene needs. The recommendations for practice are relevant for all patients.

Coleman P. (2002) Improving oral health care for the frail elderly: a review of widespread problems and best practices. *Geriatric Nursing* **23**(4):189–199.
A review of preventative measures and an oral health assessment tool for use. Some useful suggestions for enhancing oral care in cognitively impaired residents.

McGee P. (2002) Nursing with dignity. *Nursing Times* **98**(9):33–35.
This is the first in a series of nine articles relating to meeting the needs of clients from different cultural backgrounds.

Popoola MM, Jenkins L. (2005) Caring for the foot mobile: holistic foot and nail management. *Holistic Nursing Practice* **19**(5):222–227.
An interesting article that discusses how to identify fungal toenails and ingrown toenails, which are common foot problems.

Notes

12

Respiratory care

ASSESSMENT OF BREATHING AND COUNTING RESPIRATIONS

Preparation

Patient	Equipment/Environment	Nurse
• The patient should be relaxed and resting, or recent activity should be noted. • Do not inform the patient when you will be assessing breathing **PFP1**.	• Watch with a second hand.	• The hands should be clean. • Additional protective clothing may be necessary if indicated by the patient's condition (see Chapter 9).

Procedure

1. Observe the movement of the chest wall for symmetry of chest movement and whether accessory muscles are being used **PFP2**.
2. Observe the rhythm and depth of respirations.
3. Count the respirations for 60 seconds **PFP3**.
4. Observe for the following:
   - Difficulty in breathing.
   - Pain on breathing and its location.
   - Noisy respiration – whether there is any wheeze or stridor.
   - Cough – whether dry or productive.
   - Sputum – amount, colour and consistency (see page 317).
5. Observe the patient's colour for signs of cyanosis **PFP4**.

Post procedure

Patient	Nurse
• Ensure the patient is comfortable. A patient with breathing difficulties may be most comfortable sitting upright (see page 302).	• Record/chart the respiratory observations according to local policy and report any abnormalities (see Figure 1.7 for an example of charting). • Adjust the frequency of observations as necessary.

Points for practice

1. A more accurate observation is obtained if the patient is unaware that their respirations are being counted. Many nurses achieve this by pretending to be feeling the radial pulse when in fact observing the movement of the chest wall (Figure 12.1).

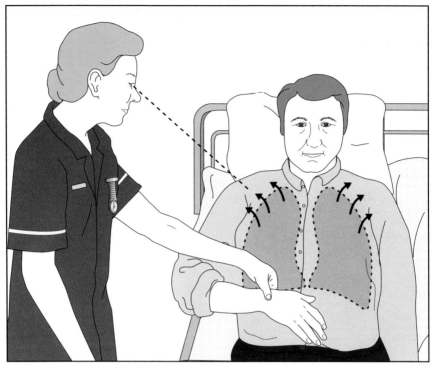

Figure 12.1 Monitoring the respiration rate while apparently counting the pulse

2. Accessory muscles are the sternocleidomastoid and trapezius muscles in the neck and shoulders. If these are being used it indicates that the patient is unable to use the diaphragm and external intercostal muscles adequately (Esmond 2001).

3. If breathing is very shallow and difficult to observe, lightly rest your hand on the patient's chest or abdomen to feel movement. The normal rate for an adult is 12–20 breaths per minute.

4. Cyanosis is a blue discoloration of the skin and mucous membranes and is most noticeable around the lips, earlobes, mouth and fingertips. In dark-skinned patients, signs of poor perfusion or cyanosis may be detected if the area around the lips or nail beds is dusky in colour.

POSITIONING THE BREATHLESS PATIENT

Preparation

Patient	Equipment/Environment	Nurse
• Explain the procedure, to gain consent and co-operation.	• Bed with adjustable backrest or electric raising mechanism.	• Two nurses may be needed.
• The patient may be anxious because of the difficulty in breathing.	• Four or five pillows.	• An apron should be worn if assisting the patient to move.
	• Bed table with brakes.	• Additional protective clothing may be necessary if indicated by the patient's condition (see Chapter 9).
	• Firm, supporting armchair.	
	• A hoist or sliding aid may be needed if the patient is unable to move up the bed unaided.	

Procedure

1. Explain to the patient exactly what is planned so that movement is reduced to a minimum.

2. Ask/assist the patient to sit forward. A second nurse may be needed to support the patient while the backrest is adjusted and the pillows are arranged **PFP1**.

3. Adjust the backrest or raise the head of the bed.

4. Arrange the pillows so that the patient feels supported. This will vary according to patient preference, but you should ensure that the lumbar region is supported **PFP1**.

5. If the foot of the bed can be raised slightly, this may help to prevent the patient slipping down.

6. For a short period, the patient may get relief by leaning forward with the forearms resting on a pillow on a bed table (Figure 12.2).

7. If able to get out of bed, the breathless patient is often most comfortable sitting in an armchair, and many prefer to sleep in this position.

Post procedure

Patient	Equipment/Environment	Nurse
• Observe for changes in respiratory pattern, cough, colour, etc. (see page 300).	• If sitting for long periods, a pressure-relieving mattress or cushion may be needed to prevent pressure ulcers **PFP2**.	• Document the care given and report any change in condition.
• Ensure drink, call bell, etc., are close to hand.		

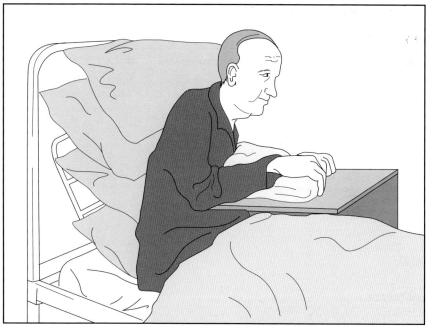

Figure 12.2 Positioning the breathless patient

Points for practice

1. When positioning the breathless patient, the aim is to maximise respiratory functioning while reducing physical effort; therefore, the patient must be comfortable and well-supported. Ensure the pillows are supporting the small of the back so that the patient does not sink into them and thus restrict chest movement.

2. Regular re-positioning is necessary to prevent pressure ulcers (see Chapter 13).

FACE MASKS AND NASAL CANNULAE

Preparation

Patient	Equipment/Environment	Nurse
• Explain the procedure, to gain co-operation and consent.	• Piped oxygen or oxygen cylinder `PFP2`.	• The hands should be clean when handling oxygen equipment.
• Prepare the patient pre-operatively if oxygen therapy is planned post-operatively.	• Oxygen tubing `PFP3`. • Prescription chart `PFP4`. • Mask or nasal cannulae as prescribed `PFP5`.	• Additional protective clothing may be necessary if indicated by the patient's condition (see Chapter 9).
• Patients and visitors must be made aware of the dangers of smoking when oxygen is being administered `PFP1`.		

Procedure

1. Except in an emergency situation, oxygen therapy must be prescribed by a doctor.

2. Turn on the oxygen flow meter and set the flow rate (Figures 12.3 & 12.4B).

3. Place the mask over the patient's nose and mouth with the elastic strap over the ears to the back of the head. Adjust the length of the strap to ensure the mask fits securely (Figure 12.4A).

4. If using nasal cannulae, place 2 cm of tubing into the nostrils; the other tubes go over the ears and either under the chin or behind the head (Figure 12.4C).

Post procedure

Patient	Equipment/Environment	Nurse
• Observe the patient's colour/perfusion and respiratory pattern.	• Tubing and masks may be reused several times for the same patient. It should be disposed of in the clinical waste when no longer required.	• Monitor respiratory pattern and rate (see page 300).
• Offer drinks or mouth care `PFP7`.	• If using an oxygen cylinder, ensure that a replacement cylinder is available when the volume indicator gauge shows a quarter full.	• Document oxygen therapy according to local policy.

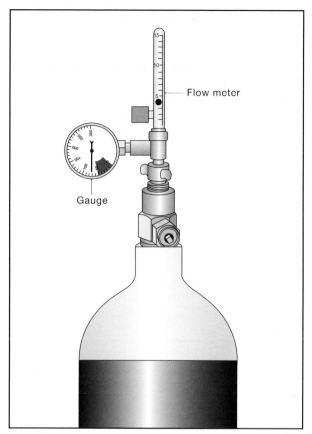

Figure 12.3 Oxygen cylinder

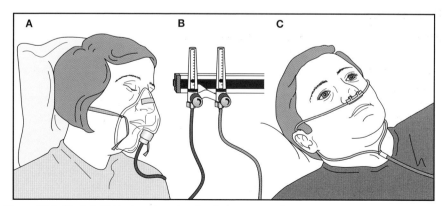

Figure 12.4 (A, B & C) Hudson-type mask, etc.

Points for practice

1. Oxygen is highly inflammable.

2. An oxygen cylinder has a black base with white shoulders and has 'oxygen' written on it (Figure 12.3).

3. Oxygen tubing may come in prepacked lengths as a continuous roll with a 'bubble' (widened portion) at regular intervals. Cut through the centre of the bubble and then further trim as necessary to ensure a secure fit onto the flow meter and mask. The length should allow freedom of movement for the patient, but not be so long that it may become kinked or touch the floor.

4. Oxygen therapy must be prescribed, except in emergency situations.

5. If a percentage of oxygen has been prescribed, a special mask that incorporates a Venturi system is used (Figure 12.5). These are colour coded and specify the flow of oxygen required to deliver 24%, 28%, 35%, 40% and 60% oxygen.

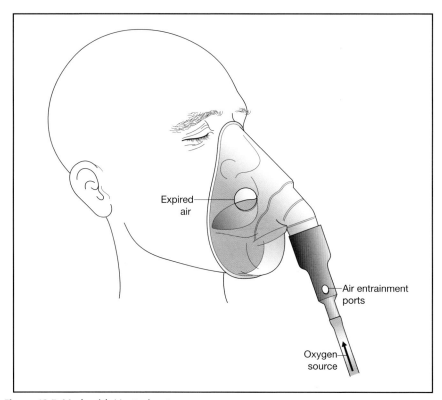

Figure 12.5 Mask with Venturi system

A Hudson mask is used to deliver a high concentration of oxygen, i.e. greater than 60%.

If nasal cannulae are used, the flow rate of the oxygen must not exceed 2 l/minute or it will damage the nasal mucosa.

6. The centre of the ball in the flow meter must sit at the level of the flow rate prescribed.

7. Oxygen therapy dries the mucous membranes of the mouth. Frequent drinks should be taken or frequent mouth care provided if the oxygen is not being humidified. Humidification should always be considered if oxygen therapy is required for prolonged periods and for patients with respiratory infections who have difficulty expectorating sputum (Esmond 2001) (see page 308).

HUMIDIFIED OXYGEN

Preparation

Patient

- Explain the procedure, to gain consent and co-operation.

Equipment/Environment

- Piped oxygen or oxygen cylinder.
- Large-bore 'elephant' tubing.
- Humidifier and water reservoir.

Nurse

- The hands should be clean and the principles of asepsis maintained when handling the water reservoir of the humidifier.

Procedure

1. Check the prescription regarding the percentage of oxygen to be administered `PFP1`.
2. Connect the humidifier to the oxygen flow meter according to the manufacturer's instructions `PFP2`.
3. Connect the wide-bore tubing to the mask and set the flow meter to the flow required to achieve the prescribed percentage of oxygen `PFP3`.
4. A fine mist should appear in the mask. Ask/assist the patient to put on the mask and adjust the retaining strap to prevent pressure on the ears. The nose part of the mask may need to be adjusted to prevent mist going into the eyes (Figure 12.6).

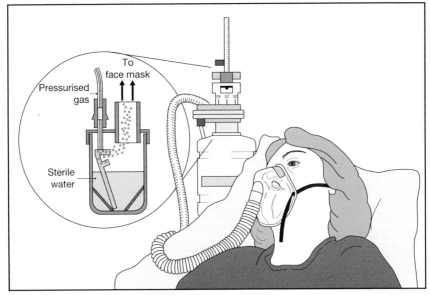

Figure 12.6 Humidified oxygen

Post procedure

Patient

- Ensure the patient is comfortable.
- The humidified oxygen may encourage the patient to cough so a sputum pot and tissues should be provided.

Equipment/Environment

- If using an oxygen cylinder, monitor the amount remaining and order a replacement when it is down to quarter full.
- Check regularly to see if water is collecting in the tubing **PFP4**.
- The water reservoir should be replaced when empty.
- The tubing and mask should be changed every 24 hours.

Nurse

- Document humidified oxygen therapy in the nursing records.

Points for practice

1. Except in an emergency situation, all oxygen therapy must be prescribed.
2. Connection will vary according to the type of humidifier. Usually it is achieved by removing the connector at the base of the flow meter, attaching the humidifier by screwing it into position.
3. It is important that the flow is set at the rate indicated to achieve the prescribed percentage. This is usually indicated on the top of the humidifier where it attaches to the flow meter. There may also be a valve adjustment, which should be turned to the correct setting.
4. Water that collects in the wide-bore tubing should be emptied or the tubing changed according to local policy.

USE OF NEBULISER

Preparation

Patient

- Explain the procedure, to gain consent and co-operation.
- The patient should be in a comfortable position, sitting upright.

Equipment/Environment

- Air or oxygen (piped or cylinder) according to prescription `PFP1`.
- Nebuliser and face mask or mouthpiece `PFP2`.
- Nebuliser solution and prescription chart `PFP3`.

Nurse

- The hands should be clean and the principles of asepsis maintained when handling the nebuliser and solution.
- Additional protective clothing may be necessary if indicated by the patient's condition (see Chapter 9).

Procedure

1. Check the nebuliser solution and the patient's identity with the prescription (page 139).
2. Unscrew the base of the nebuliser and add the solution (this is usually in a plastic ampoule that is squeezed to expel the liquid), then screw together again (Figure 12.7A).

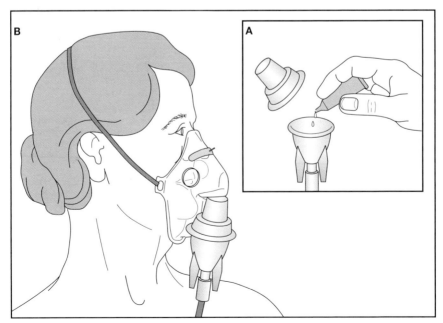

Figure 12.7 (A) Adding the nebuliser solution, (B) nebuliser therapy

3. Make sure the mouthpiece or face mask is securely attached to the nebuliser.

4. Set the flow meter on the air cylinder to 6 l/minute. A fine mist should appear in the mask and a hissing sound will be heard.

5. Ask/assist the patient to use the mouthpiece or put on the mask by placing the retaining strap over the ears and back of the head (Figure 12.7B).

Post procedure

Patient	**Equipment/Environment**	**Nurse**
• The patient should remain sitting upright until all the solution has been vaporised. This may take up to 10 minutes. • The nebuliser is likely to encourage the patient to cough, so a sputum pot and tissues should be provided.	• If the nebuliser is to be used again, it should be left clean and dry and stored in a plastic bag on the patient's locker.	• Document nebuliser therapy according to local policy. • A peak expiratory flow rate may be requested before and after the nebuliser (see page 312).

Points for practice

1. The use of air or oxygen will depend on the underlying disease process. Most patients with asthma will be prescribed oxygen, whereas those with chronic obstructive pulmonary disease (COPD) are usually prescribed their nebulisers with air. If using a cylinder, check that it is at least a quarter full. Air cylinders are grey-green in colour with black and while shoulders. Oxygen cylinders have a black base with white shoulders (see Figure 12.3).

2. Wherever possible, a mouthpiece is the preferred option as it provides better deposition of the drug into the lungs and reduces side effects (Esmond 2001). If the patient is having nebuliser therapy regularly, the mask or mouthpiece will be kept at the bedside between uses. Nebuliser therapy is usually administered two to four times per day.

3. Drugs to be nebulised (e.g. a bronchodilator) must be prescribed and this must be checked according to local policy (see page 139).

PEAK EXPIRATORY FLOW RATE

Preparation

Patient	Equipment/Environment	Nurse
• Explain the procedure, to gain consent and co-operation.	• Peak flow meter.	• The hands should be clean.
	• Disposable mouthpiece.	
	• Chart to record measurement.	
• Ideally, the patient should be standing. If the patient's condition does not allow this, they should sit as upright as possible PFP1.		
• The patient should be rested, as recent exertion may affect the accuracy of the measurement.		

Procedure

1. Attach disposable mouthpiece.
2. Set pointer on the peak flow meter to zero.
3. Instruct the patient to inhale deeply, place their lips around the mouthpiece, and holding the meter horizontally, exhale forcibly (**Figure 12.8**). Make sure that the patient's fingers do not occlude the pointer.
4. Note the measurement.
5. Repeat steps 2–4 twice more PFP2.
6. Record the highest of the three measurements (**Figure 12.9**).

Post procedure

Patient	Equipment/Environment	Nurse
• Ensure the patient is comfortable.	• The disposable mouthpiece may be reused for the same patient. Keep dry and protected from dust.	• Record measurement. Pre- and post-nebuliser recordings should be recorded in different colours to differentiate between them (Figure 12.9).
• Peak expiratory flow rate measurement may be required before and after a nebuliser PFP3.		• Report any abnormality or significant variation from previous recordings PFP4.
		• Report any distress caused to the patient by this activity.

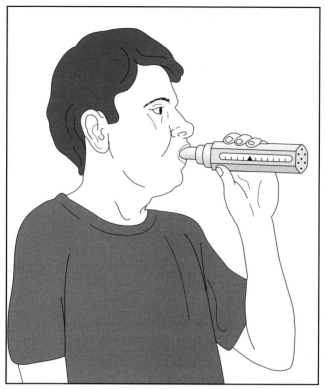

Figure 12.8 Peak flow rate measurement

Points for practice

1. The patient should adopt the position they usually adopt when recording peak expiratory flow rate, but sitting upright or standing is best (Higgins 2005).

2. If the procedure causes the patient distress (e.g. excessive coughing or wheezing), ask the patient to do one recording only. Document this on the chart.

3. If the peak expiratory flow rate is to be measured after a nebuliser, this should be done 30 minutes afterwards (Higgins 2005).

4. The peak expiratory flow rate varies according to age, sex and stature. It is measured in litres per minute.

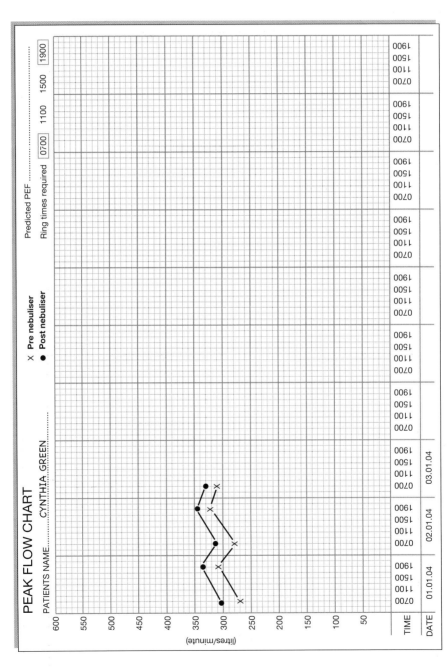

Figure 12.9 Peak flow chart

PULSE OXIMETRY (OXYGEN SATURATION)

Preparation

Patient	Equipment/Environment	Nurse
• Explain the procedure, to gain co-operation and consent.	• Pulse oximeter PFP1. • Sensor appropriate to patient's size and condition. • Alcohol-impregnated swabs.	• The hands should be clean. • Additional protective clothing may be necessary if indicated by the patient's condition (see Chapter 9).

Procedure

1. Assess the patient's peripheral circulation in order to choose an appropriate sensor. The most usual are those that clip onto the patient's finger, although sensors that clip onto the ears or adhesive nasal sensors are available (Figure 12.10).

2. Before applying the sensor, clean the skin with an alcohol-impregnated swab or soap and water and ensure that the skin is clean and dry.

3. If using a finger sensor, remove false nails or nail polish, as this could give a false reading PFP2. Avoid placing the finger probe on the same arm as a blood pressure cuff as the reading will be inaccurate during inflation of the cuff.

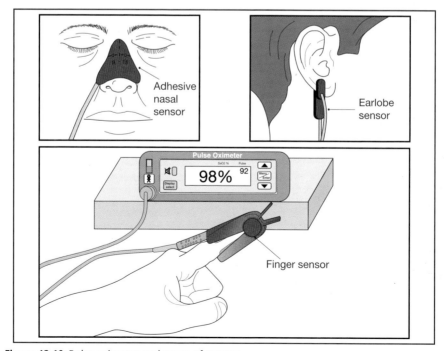

Figure 12.10 Pulse oximeter and types of sensors

4. Attach the sensor according to the manufacturer's instructions then plug the cable into the pulse oximeter and turn on the machine.

5. Observe waveform fluctuations to ensure that the pulse waveform is registering **PFP3**.

6. Set alarm limits on pulse oximeter if not pre-set by manufacturer.

7. If continuous oxygen saturation measurements are required, change the sensor site every 4 hours to prevent pressure damage or irritation from adhesive sensors.

8. If intermittent oxygen saturations are being measured, remove the sensor between readings.

Post procedure

Patient	Equipment/Environment	Nurse
• Ensure patient is comfortable. • If using adhesive sensors remove any traces of adhesive with acetone.	• Unplug pulse oximeter and store in equipment storage area. • Store sensor cable as per manufacturer's recommendations.	• Document oxygen saturation measurement in the nursing records, noting whether the patient is receiving oxygen therapy (see page 304). • Document the state of the patient's perfusion noting any changes in mental status or colour of the skin. • Report any change/ abnormal findings immediately.

Points for practice

1. The pulse oximeter is used to measure oxygen saturation (SpO_2) levels. The normal level is 95–99% (Clark & Giuliano 2006). The pulse oximeter will also show the pulse rate, but it is important to feel the patient's pulse rate to be able to monitor the rhythm and strength of the pulse.

2. Patients with jaundice may give falsely high readings due to high serum bilirubin levels. If the patient has recently had any investigations that involve the injection of radio-opaque dyes, then this may cause spurious readings (Higgins 2005).

3. Some models of pulse oximeter do not show a pulse waveform, just a digital readout.

OBSERVATION OF SPUTUM

Preparation

Patient	Equipment/Environment	Nurse
• Explain the procedure, to gain consent and co-operation. • Ensure privacy – the patient may be distressed or embarrassed at having to expectorate.	• Disposable sputum carton with lid. • Tissues. • Clinical waste bag.	• Gloves should be worn if the patient needs assistance with expectoration, use of tissues, etc. • Additional protective clothing may be necessary if indicated by the patient's condition (see Chapter 9).

Procedure

1. Expectoration will be easier if the patient is sitting up, supported by pillows, or is sitting in an armchair.
2. Encourage the patient to expectorate into the sputum pot rather than swallowing the sputum **PFP1**. 'Huffing' may help the patient to expectorate.
3. Observe the sputum for the following:
   - Quantity.
   - Consistency: whether watery, frothy or tenacious (sticky).
   - Colour: white – mucus; yellow/green – pus (infected); red – fresh blood (haemoptysis).
   - Odour: foul-smelling sputum may indicate a lung abscess.

Post procedure

Patient	Equipment/Environment	Nurse
• The patient may feel very tired after a bout of coughing. • A mouthwash or drink should be offered.	• Remove used sputum carton, observe, and then close the lid tightly and discard in the yellow clinical waste bag. • Provide patient with clean sputum carton.	• Remove gloves and wash hands. • Document the amount and nature of the sputum.

Points for practice

1. The assistance of a physiotherapist may be necessary to teach the patient how to breathe deeply and expectorate without strain rather than coughing ineffectively.

OBTAINING A SPUTUM SPECIMEN

Preparation

Patient	Equipment/Environment	Nurse
• Explain the procedure and the number of specimens required PFP1.	• Universal specimen pot. • Plastic specimen bag and laboratory request form. • Drinking water and mouthwash. • Tissues.	• Gloves should be worn if the patient needs assistance with expectoration, use of tissues, etc. • Additional protective clothing may be necessary if indicated by the patient's condition (see Chapter 9)

Procedure

1. Ask the patient to rinse their mouth thoroughly with water PFP2.
2. Ask/assist the patient to expectorate into the sterile pot PFP3.
3. Seal the lid and complete the label with the date, patient's full name, hospital number, ward and type of specimen.
4. Place the pot and the laboratory request form in a plastic specimen bag and dispatch to the laboratory straight away PFP4.

Post procedure

Patient	Equipment/Environment	Nurse
• Ensure the patient is comfortable and offer a mouthwash and/or tissues as appropriate.	• Dispose of any waste appropriately.	• Document that the specimen has been obtained. • Note colour, smell and consistency.

Points for practice

1. Three consecutive early-morning specimens may be requested for acid-fast bacilli (tuberculosis) or for cytology (malignant cells).
2. The mouth should be rinsed with water (not mouthwash) before expectoration, to reduce contamination of the specimen with food.
3. When obtaining the specimen it is important to ensure that it is mucoid or mucopurulent, which indicates that it is sputum and not just saliva (Wilson 2006).
4. Sputum specimens must be sent to the laboratory immediately as respiratory pathogens will not survive for long periods. If refrigerated for more than 12 hours *Haemophilus influenzae* and *Streptococcus pneumoniae* may die and gram-negative organisms over grow in the specimen (Wilson 2006).

ORAL SUCTIONING

Preparation

Patient	Equipment/Environment	Nurse
• Explain the procedure, to gain consent and co-operation.	• Suction machine (if piped suction is not available).	• The hands must be washed and dried thoroughly.
• The patient requiring oral suctioning may be semi-conscious or unconscious. If so, they should be positioned on their side, facing the nurse PFP1.	• Suction tubing and oral sucker, e.g. Yankauer sucker (**Figure 12.11**).	• An apron and gloves should be worn.
	• Sterile distilled water PFP2.	• Goggles will be required if airborne secretions are likely.

Procedure

1. Switch on the suction machine and attach the tubing and oral sucker, ensuring a good fit to prevent loss of suction pressure PFP3.

2. If able to co-operate, ask the patient to open their mouth.

3. The oral sucker may have a hole which when occluded by your thumb enables suction to be applied. If the oral sucker has no suction-control mechanism, kink the suction tubing so that suction is not applied until required.

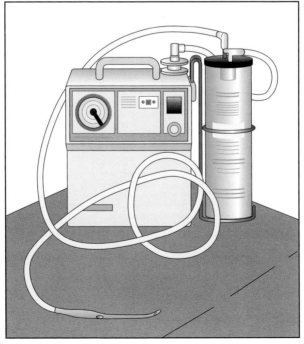

Figure 12.11 Suction machine with Yankauer sucker attached

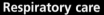
4. Gently insert the oral sucker into the mouth, taking care not to make the patient 'gag' by inserting it too far.

5. Apply suction, moving the sucker to all parts of the mouth as necessary.

6. Release suction and remove oral sucker from the mouth.

Post procedure

Patient	Equipment/Environment	Nurse
• Ensure the patient is comfortable.	• Clean the oral sucker and suction tubing by suctioning sterile water through it until all traces of sputum have gone.	• Remove gloves and apron and wash hands.
• Mouth care may be required following oral suctioning (see page 285).		• Document oral suctioning, noting the amount and appearance of the secretions.
	• The oral sucker may be used again on the same patient providing it is left clean and covered by a plastic bag between uses. The sucker and tubing should be replaced every 24 hours.	
	• Replace the cap on the bottle of sterile distilled water.	
	• If the suction machine has a reusable bottle, this should be emptied at least every 24 hours. Goggles should be worn when emptying it. If it has a disposable sealed container, this does not need to be emptied but sealed and discarded when full or when the patient no longer requires suctioning.	

Points for practice

1. Oral suctioning may be required by patients who are able to cough, but are too weak to expectorate. It may also be necessary during cardiopulmonary resuscitation and in unconscious patients if there are copious secretions.

2. The sterile distilled water is used to clean the suction tubing after use and must be kept closed to discourage bacterial growth. The bottle must be changed every 24 hours. If poured into a bowl, the bowl must be kept clean and dry when not in use.

3. There is little supporting evidence for correct suction pressure for oral suctioning, but it is suggested that 20 kPa is the maximum pressure required (Bennet 2003).

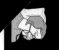

CARE OF A TRACHEOSTOMY

Preparation

Patient	Equipment/Environment	Nurse
• Explain the procedure, to gain consent and co-operation.	• Sterile dressing pack containing gloves.	• The hands must be washed and dried thoroughly.
• Tracheostomy care is easier if the patient is recumbent or semi-recumbent in bed.	• Extra gauze swabs may be needed.	• An apron should be worn.
	• Dressing trolley or other suitable surface.	• Two nurses will be needed when changing the tapes (one to hold the tube).
	• Keyhole dressing according to local policy.	
	• Two tracheostomy tapes.	
	• Cleansing solution according to local policy **PFP1**.	
	• Tracheal dilators **PFP2**.	
	• Alcohol hand-rub or hand washing facilities.	
	• Scissors to cut tapes.	

Procedure

1. It is a good idea to perform suction (see page 325) prior to the dressing change, to minimise the risk of coughing and dislodgement of the tube.

2. Prepare the trolley and equipment (see page 258).

3. Raise the bed to a safe working height. Remove any humidification/oxygen apparatus from the tracheostomy site, but leave the tapes tied **PFP3**.

4. Wash your hands or clean them using alcohol hand-rub.

5. Open the dressing pack, keyhole dressing and cleansing solution, and use the yellow waste bag as a 'glove' to remove the old dressing (see page 260).

6. Attach the waste bag to the side of the trolley nearest the patient. Put on the sterile gloves.

7. Use gauze swabs and cleansing solution to clean around the tracheostomy as necessary. Use gauze swabs to gently dry the site.

8. Apply the keyhole dressing (**Figure 12.12A**).

9. With a second nurse holding the tube in position, cut the tapes, taking care not to cut the pilot tube if it is a cuffed tracheostomy tube, and remove the old tapes **PFP4**.

10. Fold one new tape so that there is a long end (about two-thirds of the length of the tape) and a short end (about one-third of the length of the tape). Thread the folded part through the hole in the flange on the tracheostomy

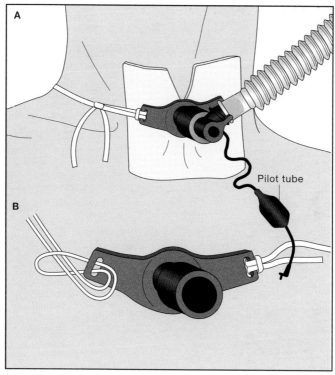

Figure 12.12 (A) 'Keyhole' tracheostomy dressing, (B) threading the tapes through the loop

tube (**Figure 12.12B**), create a loop and thread the rest of the tape through it to secure it. Repeat for the other tape.

11. Pass the long end of each tape behind the patient's neck and tie each securely to the short end on the other side. A secure knot, not a bow, must be used to prevent it becoming loose. It should be just possible to slip a finger between the tape and the patient's neck.

12. The long end of the tapes may be threaded through a foam protector before tieing, to prevent them cutting into the patient's neck.

Post procedure

Patient	Equipment/Environment	Nurse
• Replace any humidification/oxygen apparatus. • Ensure the patient is comfortable and there is no respiratory distress.	• Discard all clinical waste appropriately.	• Remove apron and wash hands. • Document the dressing change, noting the appearance of the tracheostomy site.

Points for practice

1. The cleansing solution may vary according to local policy, but 0.9% sodium chloride is usually sufficient.

2. Tracheal dilators should always be kept by the patient's bedside in case the tracheostomy is dislodged. However, once the tracheostomy is well established, the opening is unlikely to close if the tube is temporarily removed.

3. If the patient is on a ventilator, this must not be disconnected during the dressing change. The second nurse will be needed to support the tubing, etc., to facilitate the dressing change.

4. Two nurses are needed to safely change the tracheostomy tapes, so that one can hold the tube in position to prevent dislodgement if the patient coughs or moves unexpectedly.

TRACHEAL SUCTIONING

Preparation

Patient	Equipment/Environment	Nurse
• Explain the procedure, to gain consent and co-operation.	• Suction machine (if piped suction is not available).	• Wash and dry hands thoroughly.
• The patient will have an endotracheal (ET) tube or tracheostomy PFP1.	• Suction tubing.	• Wear a non-sterile glove on your non-dominant hand and an apron PFP3.
	• Suction catheters with suction-control mechanism.	• Goggles PFP4.
	• Sterile distilled water PFP2.	
	• Supply of single sterile gloves PFP3.	
	• Yellow clinical waste bag/bin.	

Procedure

1. Turn on the suction machine and test the suction pressure PFP5.

2. Open the suction-control end of a suction catheter, but leave it in its packet. Attach the end to the suction tubing, ensuring a good fit so that suction pressure is not lost.

3. Place the tubing and suction catheter (still in its packet) in a convenient position ready for use.

4. Open a sterile glove and put it on your dominant hand.

5. With your non-dominant hand, remove any humidifying/oxygen apparatus from the ET tube/tracheostomy PFP6.

6. With the same hand, pick up the suction tubing and carefully pull the suction catheter out of its packet.

7. As the suction catheter emerges, take hold of it in your sterile-gloved hand, about halfway down the catheter. Do not allow the catheter to touch anything.

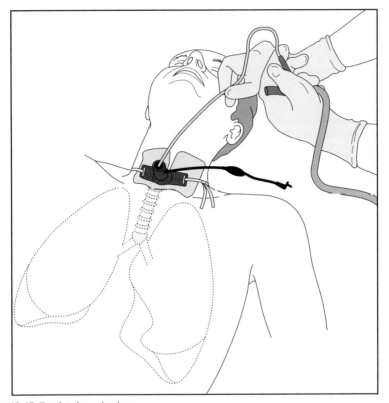

Figure 12.13 Tracheal suctioning

8. Insert the suction catheter into the ET tube/tracheostomy and, after warning the patient, advance it until it reaches the bifurcation of the right and left main bronchi (**Figure 12.13**). This will make the patient cough PFP7.

9. When the patient coughs, withdraw the suction catheter 1–2 cm and then apply suction by occluding the suction-control apparatus with the thumb of your non-dominant hand PFP8.

10. Continue to apply suction and gradually withdraw the catheter, rolling it between your fingers and thumb as you do so.

11. Remove the catheter from the ET tube/tracheostomy and wrap it around the fingers of your sterile-gloved hand. Remove the glove, turning it inside out with the catheter contained within it.

12. Disconnect the catheter from the suction tubing and discard.

13. Repeat as necessary using a new catheter and sterile glove each time PFP9.

Post procedure

Patient	Equipment/Environment	Nurse
• Replace any humidification/oxygen apparatus. • Ensure the patient is comfortable and breathing has returned to its usual rate.	• Clean the suction tubing by suctioning sterile water through it until all traces of sputum have gone. The tubing should be replaced every 24 hours. • Attach a suction catheter and leave it in its packet ready for next use. • Replace the cap on the bottle of sterile distilled water. • If the suction machine has a disposable sealed container, this does not need to be emptied, but sealed and discarded when full or when the patient no longer requires suctioning. If it has a reusable bottle, this should be emptied at least every 24 hours. Goggles should be worn when emptying it as there is a high risk of splashing (see Chapter 9).	• Remove gloves and apron and wash hands. • Document suctioning, noting the amount and appearance of the secretions.

Points for practice

1. The need for suctioning should be determined by a thorough assessment including auscultation of the chest (Day et al 2002).

2. The sterile distilled water is used to clean the suction tubing after use and must be kept closed to discourage bacterial growth. The bottle must be changed every 24 hours. If the water is poured into a bowl, the bowl must be kept clean and dry when not in use.

3. A new single sterile glove is used with each suction catheter. A non-sterile glove should be worn on your non-dominant hand to prevent contact with tracheal secretions when the suction-control apparatus is occluded with your thumb. If the catheter does not have an integral suction-control mechanism, a 'Y' connector may be inserted to serve the purpose.

4. Some authors recommend that goggles are worn because of the risk of airborne secretions when the patient coughs (Day et al 2002).

5. Suction pressure should be 10–20 kPa (Day et al 2002).

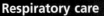
6. If the patient is on a ventilator, the top of the ET tube/tracheostomy should be removed at the last minute and replaced immediately after each suctioning. Suction should be performed swiftly, no more than 10–15 seconds, as the patient is unable to breathe unaided. A guide is to hold your own breath as you insert the catheter and aim to complete suctioning by the time you need to breathe again.

7. When the suction catheter touches the tracheal wall, the patient will cough, sometimes violently. Patients find this unpleasant and often distressing, but it is important to induce coughing to prevent stasis of secretions in the lungs.

8. The suction catheter should be rolled between the fingers as it is withdrawn, to facilitate the removal of secretions and to prevent high pressure being applied to any part of the tracheal wall. The tips of most suction catheters are designed to minimise this.

9. Suctioning can be repeated until the ET tube/tracheostomy is clear of secretions and the breathing sounds clear. However, this may be distressing and so it may be necessary to allow time for the patient to rest during the procedure. No more than three suction passes should be made at any one time.

INSERTION AND MANAGEMENT OF CHEST DRAINS

Preparation

Patient

- Explain the procedure, to gain co-operation and consent.
- Explain positioning of the tube and subsequent limitations to mobility.
- Explain the importance of not raising the bottle higher than the patient's chest PFP1.
- Ask/assist the patient to move into the required position – usually sitting forward resting on a table for support.
- Ensure privacy and dignity are maintained throughout.

Equipment/Environment

- Dressing trolley or clean surface.
- Sterile chest drain insertion pack or dressing pack.
- Hypoallergenic adhesive tape.
- Goggles, sterile gown and gloves for doctor.
- Antiseptic skin-cleansing solution according to local policy.
- Local anaesthetic as prescribed.
- Syringes and needles for administration of local anaesthetic.
- Sterile disposable scalpel.
- Suture material (usually silk) for purse-string and retaining suture.
- Sterile chest drain and introducer/trochar.
- Sterile drainage equipment (usually disposable) and sterile water.
- Two tubing clamps PFP2.
- Sharps bin.

Nurse

- The nurse's role during chest drain insertion is to observe and support the patient and assist the doctor.
- Record the patient's blood pressure, pulse, respiratory rate and oxygen saturation as baseline measurements.
- Wash and dry hands thoroughly.
- Put on apron. Additional protective clothing may be necessary if indicated by the patient's condition (see Chapter 9).

Procedure

1. Administer sedative or analgesic (if prescribed) 20 minutes before the procedure.

2. Maintaining the principles of asepsis, assemble the drainage equipment and add the water. Make sure that the tube to be attached to the chest drain tubing is 4–5 cm below the water level (Figure 12.14) PFP3.

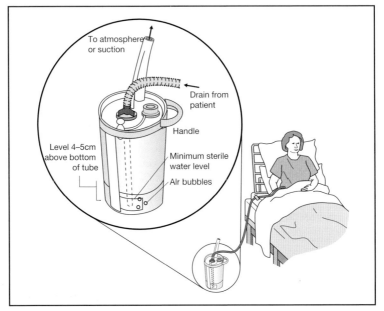

To atmosphere
or suction

Drain from
patient

Handle

Level 4–5cm
above bottom
of tube

Minimum sterile
water level

Air bubbles

Figure 12.14 Underwater seal chest drain

3. Open the sterile pack and add the sterile gown, gloves, syringe, scalpel and suture material.

4. Pour the antiseptic skin-cleansing solution into a gallipot. The doctor will now put on the goggles, sterile gown and gloves.

5. When requested by the doctor, open the sterile needle for attachment to the syringe and hold the ampoule of local anaesthetic for the doctor to check and then draw into the syringe. This will then be used to numb the proposed insertion site.

6. When requested by the doctor, open the packaging of the chest drain and introducer/trochar. The trochar will be placed inside the chest drain and then inserted into the chest wall.

7. During insertion of the chest drain observe the patient for signs of discomfort or respiratory distress.

8. Once the chest drain is inserted it should be attached to the drainage bottle immediately. The tubing may be clamped to prevent further lung collapse prior to attachment to the drainage bottle. Once securely attached, remove clamp.

9. The drain is then sutured in place and a purse-string suture inserted by the doctor **PFP4**. The drain should be further secured to the chest wall with adhesive tape and the site covered with a dry dressing **PFP5**.

10. Check that the drainage system is functioning by observing for swinging movement of water in the tubing as the patient breathes. There should be bubbling in the water with respiration in the case of

a pneumothorax, and drainage of blood into the bottle in the case of a haemothorax PFP6.

11. If suction has been prescribed, the suction tubing is attached to the short tube in the bottle, the one that does not touch the water PFP7.

Post procedure

Patient	Equipment/Environment	Nurse
• Ensure that the patient is comfortable and that the tubing of the chest drain is not pulling or kinked. A chest X-ray will be required to confirm the position of the chest drain. • Patients should be encouraged to mobilise and sit up where possible. Deep breathing and coughing promote pleural drainage PFP8.	• Discard all clinical waste appropriately. • Discard needles, scalpel and the chest drain introducer into the sharps bin.	• Remove apron and wash hands. • Record the patient's blood pressure, pulse, respiratory rate and oxygen saturation at least 4 hourly. • Document the chest drain insertion and, if applicable, the amount of suction required. • Monitor drainage, whether the fluid level is 'swinging' and any air leak/bubbling.

Points for practice

1. The drainage bottle should always be kept below the level of the patient's chest to prevent siphoning of fluid into the pleural space (Thorn 2006).

2. Chest drain tubes should only be clamped if accidental disconnection occurs or when bottles are being changed. Unnecessary clamping of tubes may cause a tension pneumothorax.

3. The end of the long tube in the bottle must be underwater to prevent air being drawn into the lungs during inspiration. It should be no more than 4–5 cm beneath the water level as this may make expansion of the lung more difficult.

4. If more than one drain has been inserted, make sure they are clearly labelled (e.g. basal and apical).

5. The tubing can be secured to the patient's clothing by wrapping tape around the tubing and placing a safety pin through the tape. This can prevent kinks in the tubing, which will prevent drainage.

6. To facilitate measurement of the rate of drainage, a piece of tape placed vertically next to the calibrated scale of the bottle can be marked at suitable intervals. If the bottle requires changing because it is nearly full, a new bottle

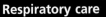

should be prepared as in procedure point 2. The chest drain should be double clamped close to the chest and the tubing disconnected from the full bottle. The new bottle is then attached, ensuring that there is an underwater seal prior to unclamping the chest tube. The full bottle should be emptied (goggles should be worn) and discarded in the clinical waste. The amount of drainage should be recorded.

7. A suction pressure of 5kPa is usually used (Thorn 2006). Do not turn off the suction without disconnecting the tubing from the chest drain as this has an effect similar to the tube being clamped and may cause a tension pneumothorax.

8. Take care that the drainage bottles are not damaged when raising or lowering the bed.

CHEST DRAIN REMOVAL

Preparation

Patient	Equipment/Environment	Nurse
• Explain the procedure, to gain consent and co-operation.	• Dressing trolley or clean work surface.	• Two nurses are required for this procedure.
• Instruct the patient to practise deep breathing and holding their breath **PFP1**.	• Sterile dressing pack containing gloves.	• The hands should be washed and dried thoroughly.
	• Extra pair of gloves for the assisting nurse.	• Aprons should be worn.
• Ask/assist the patient to adopt an upright position which is comfortable.	• Sterile dressing towel.	• Additional protective clothing may be necessary if indicated by the patient's condition (see Chapter 9).
	• Skin-cleansing solution according to local policy **PFP2**.	
• Ensure privacy.	• Sterile dressing to cover site.	• Both nurses should wear goggles.
	• Sterile stitch cutter.	
	• Alcohol hand-rub or hand washing facilities.	
	• Large clinical waste bag.	
	• Sharps bin.	

Procedure

1. Administer any prescribed analgesic or sedative **PFP3**.

2. Take the equipment to the bedside and raise the bed to an appropriate height to avoid stooping.

3. Maintaining the principles of asepsis, open the dressing pack and pour the cleansing solution into a gallipot or fluid tray. Open the stitch cutter and dressing onto the sterile field.

4. Loosen the dressing around the drain site but do not remove.

5. Wash your hands or clean them using alcohol hand-rub.

6. Using the waste disposal bag as a 'glove', remove the dressing (see page 260).

7. Put on gloves and clean around the drain site to remove any dried blood or exudate that may impede removal of the drain.

8. Cut the knot at the loose end of the purse-string suture so that the ends are free (**Figure 12.15**). Cut and remove the suture holding the drain in place (see page 264).

9. Ask the assisting nurse to put on gloves and to tie the purse-string suture loosely **PFP4**.

10. Instruct the patient to take two deep breaths and hold it (this should have been practised beforehand).

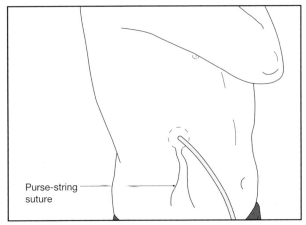

Purse-string
suture

Figure 12.15 Purse-string suture – this is pulled tight and tied as the drain is removed

11. When the patient is holding their breath, the nurse quickly and smoothly removes the chest drain. The assisting nurse pulls the purse-string suture tight and ties it with a double knot. Speed is essential.

12. On completion, instruct the patient to breathe normally.

13. Ask the assisting nurse to disconnect the chest drain tubing and discard it in the clinical waste bag **PFP5**.

14. Clean any fluid or exudate from the drain site and cover it with a dry dressing.

Post procedure

Patient	Equipment/Environment	Nurse
• Ensure the patient is comfortable **PFP6**.	• Dispose of all waste and equipment appropriately.	• Remove gloves, apron and goggles and wash hands.
• Instruct the patient to report any breathlessness/ difficulty in breathing.	• Remember to measure and record the final fluid drainage.	• Record chest drain removal in the patient's records.
• A chest X-ray may be ordered following removal of the chest drain.	• The chest drain bottle and tubing is usually disposable and can be discarded in the clinical waste. If it is not disposable, it should be returned to the sterile services department according to local policy.	

Points for practice

1. One of the main complications of chest drain removal is recurrent pneumothorax. The risk of this occurring increases if the patient breathes in whilst the drain is being removed (Bruce et al 2006).

2. The skin-cleansing solution used may vary according to local policy, but 0.9% sodium chloride is usually sufficient.

3. The doctor may prescribe analgesia or a sedative prior to chest drain removal; this should be given at least 20 minutes before the procedure. Some units now use entonox during the procedure.

4. If the drain was attached to suction, this should be disconnected before chest drain removal.

5. If two chest drains are connected to one bottle, clamp each drain close to the patient's chest and disconnect the tubing from the bottle prior to removal.

6. The purse-string suture can be removed after 5 days.

References and further reading

Bennett C. (2003) Nursing the breathless patient. *Nursing Standard* **17**(17):45–53.

A useful article giving an overview of causes of breathlessness; methods of oxygen administration; an overview of nebuliser therapy; the principles of correct inhaler technique and how to perform oropharyngeal and nasopharyngeal suctioning.

Bruce E, Howard R, Franck L. (2006) Chest drain removal pain and its management: literature review. *Journal of Clinical Nursing* **15**:145–154.

An extensive review of the evidence in relation to pain management for chest drain removal.

Clark A, Giuliano K. (2006) Pulse oximetry revisited: 'But his O_2 Sat was Normal!'. *Clinical Nurse Specialist* **20**(6):268–272.

A very good article explaining exactly what pulse oximetry measures and its limitations. Issues learned from legal cases are highlighted and discussed.

Day T, Farnell S, Haynes S, Wainwright S, Wilson-Barnett J. (2002) Tracheal suctioning: an exploration of nurses' knowledge and competence in acute and high dependency ward areas. *Journal of Advanced Nursing* **39**(1):35–45.

The main purpose of this study is to highlight nurses' knowledge in relation to tracheal suctioning; however, it identifies good practice and the evidence base for this.

Esmond G. (2001) *Respiratory nursing.* Baillière Tindall, Edinburgh.

This book provides a comprehensive resource for all aspects of respiratory nursing from the relevant A&P and respiratory assessment to smoking cessation, respiratory medication, support techniques and oxygen therapy to nutrition, pulmonary rehabilitation and end-stage management of respiratory disease.

Higgins D. (2005) Pulse oximetry. *Nursing Times* **101**(6):34–35.

A useful overview of related physiology, indications for pulse oximetry, choice of sites and the uses and limitations of pulse oximetry.

Higgins D. (2005) Measuring PEFR. *Nursing Times* **101**(10):32–33.

This article discusses the recent changes to the scale used for peak expiratory flow rate (PEFR) measurement, factors that influence it and the procedure itself.

Thorn M. (2006) Chest drains: a practical guide. *British Journal of Cardiac Nursing* 1(4):180–185.

A good overview of the indications for and principles of chest-drain management.

Jevon P, Ewens B. (2001) Assessment of a breathless patient. *Nursing Standard* **15**(16):48–50.

This comprehensive article discusses a systematic approach to the assessment of breathless patients and outlines the indications for oxygen therapy, different methods of delivery and the nursing management of patients receiving oxygen therapy. It explains the terminology used to describe respiratory disorders, the nursing required for the breathless patient and how to detect a deteriorating patient. It is part of the Continuing Professional Development series and so encourages you to reflect on your own practice and experience.

Kenward G, Hodgetts T, Castle N. (2001) Time to put the R back into TPR. *Nursing Times* 97(40):32–33.

This article emphasises the importance of counting and observing the patient's respirations as they are often the first indication that the patient is becoming unwell.

13

Immobility and associated problems

MOVING AND HANDLING

Employers' responsibilities

The implementation of a number of European Directives in 1992 led to important changes in health and safety requirements in relation to manual handling and moving. These directives stipulate that employers have a duty to ensure the safety of all employees involved in manual handling and moving activities. Employers are required to make a thorough assessment and implement measures to avoid risk. Where risk is unavoidable, they must take steps to minimise it. Employers also have a responsibility to make equipment and appropriate training available to all staff.

Employees' responsibilities

Employees have a responsibility to obey 'reasonable and lawful' instructions and to act with 'reasonable care and skill'. Thus, employees have a responsibility to attend training sessions provided by employers and to use equipment and handling aids according to the manufacturers' instructions. They also have a responsibility to inform the employers of any work situation that may require employees to work in a way that is dangerous to their health and safety. Although employers have a duty to perform risk assessments, employees equally have a responsibility to bring such situations to the employers' attention.

Safer-handling policies

Many hospitals and other institutions are working towards safer-handling or no-lifting policies. This requires the proper training and regular updating of all staff in the use of mechanical lifting equipment such as hoists, as well as sliding transfer aids and other equipment and techniques. Description of the techniques involved is beyond the scope of this book, but there are a number of principles that may be applied to any handling situation.

Principles of safe handling

- Assess the situation. Is it necessary? Would the use of equipment be safer and more effective?
- Communicate clearly, so that all involved know what to expect.
- Avoid tensing the muscles.
- Adopt a stable stance – this usually means having your feet about a hip-width apart.
- Keep your knees 'soft' (slightly bent).
- Keep the load as close to your body as possible – avoid stretching.
- Keep your back in the natural alignment and avoid twisting or bending sideways.

Risk assessment

In the UK, accident prevention is regulated by the Health and Safety at Work Act of 1974. In 1992, specific regulations in relation to moving and handling were introduced in the form of a European Directive, 'The Manual Handling Operations Regulations 1992'. The Health and Safety Executive (HSE 1992) then issued guidance on the regulations and everyone involved in manual handling operations, not just those in hospitals and nursing homes, has to comply with the HSE guidelines.

Under these guidelines it is the employer's responsibility to ensure that their employees are not at risk of injury from manual handling and to implement a policy and code of practice for the workplace that are based on advice from experts in occupational health and ergonomics. They must also employ a 'competent' person, such as a back care advisor, and carry out formal handling assessments that look at: the task, the individual nurse or carer, the load and the environment. These are important categories to remember because nurses also need to consider them in their risk assessments; the acronym TILE will help you to remember. You need to consider the following before every moving and handling activity:

Task

- Is it necessary? Can the patient move themselves or would the use of equipment be safer and more effective?
- Do you need help and/or equipment?
- Does it involve stooping, bending or twisting? If the answer is yes then you must find another way to do it.
- Is there enough time so that neither you nor the patient is rushing? For example, if the patient wants the toilet urgently it may be better to get them there quickly in a wheelchair and encourage them to walk back.

Individual nurse or carer

- What are your own capabilities? (strength, state of health, knowledge and training).
- Is your clothing appropriate? (freedom of movement).
- Are your shoes appropriate? (low heel, non-slip sole and securely fastened).
- Long hair should be tied back so that it does not fall in your face and distract you or the patient.
- Jewellery should not be worn as this may scratch the patient.
- If you are working with another nurse or carer it is best if you are of a similar height, if at all possible.

Load (Patient)

- Diagnosis/condition of the patient – is the patient 'allowed' to mobilise?
- Ability of the patient – can the patient balance, weight bear on one or both legs, etc.?
- If the patient is walking, has the patient got suitable footwear? Slippers are rarely supportive; outdoor shoes are better.
- Does the patient use any aids to mobility such as a walking stick or Zimmer frame?

- Is the patient able to understand and co-operate, e.g. are there hearing problems, language, poor sight, etc.?
- Is the patient in pain? This could lead to sudden unexpected movement and so analgesics should be administered and time allowed for this to take effect.
- Are there any intravenous infusions, drains, catheters, plaster cast, etc., to consider?

Environment

- Is there enough space to move freely without twisting or bending?
- Is the floor free of obstacles such as training wires, rugs, steps, etc.?
- Is the floor dry and not slippery?
- Is the equipment/furniture working properly, especially the brakes, height adjustment, etc.?
- Is there adequate light to see what you are doing?
- Is the temperature ambient? Being very hot makes us feel weak and very cold makes us tense our muscles.

RISK ASSESSMENT OF PRESSURE ULCERS

Principles

Pressure ulcers have long been seen as costly both in terms of patients' health and in cost to the health service. In assessing patients' susceptibility to developing pressure ulcers a number of factors must be taken into consideration. These are generally grouped into two categories: external factors and internal factors.

External factors

- **Pressure** is the most important factor and occurs when the soft tissue of the body is compressed between a bony prominence and a hard surface.

- **Shear** occurs when the soft tissues and the skeleton move, but the skin does not, e.g. sliding down the bed.

- **Friction** occurs when two surfaces rub together and the top layer of the skin is scraped off.

Internal factors

- Physical factors include the patients' general health, sensory impairment, nutrition and hydration status, level of mobility, skin condition, previous history of pressure damage and restfulness/restlessness.

- Medical/surgical factors consider patients' cardiovascular system, level of consciousness, level of pain, continence status, medications, surgery, acute, chronic or terminal illness, specific predisposing diseases, infections and allergies.

- Psychological factors incorporate an assessment of patients' mental and emotional status that may affect sleep or motivation.

- Lifestyle factors include smoking and weight and build.

- Unchangeable factors are those such as age.

In order to provide consistent information and enable nurses to plan appropriate prevention strategies a number of assessment tools have been developed (e.g. Norton et al 1975, Waterlow 2005). These assessment tools differ, but most consider the majority of factors outlined above. What is important is that the nurse uses clinical judgement in conjunction with the chosen assessment tool as it is often the existence of a combination of factors that increases patients' susceptibility to pressure ulcer formation.

Assessing the patient

Patients should receive an initial and ongoing risk assessment within 6 hours of admission in the first episode of care (NICE 2005). Assessment of the patient should address the following:

Physical factors

In combination with an assessment of patients' general health prior to admission to hospital, a thorough nutritional assessment should be undertaken using a recognised tool, such as the Malnutrition Universal Screening Tool (MUST) (see page 110). Patients who have a diet lacking in vitamin C, proteins and minerals are more susceptible to pressure ulcer development. Reduced nutritional status impairs the elasticity of the skin and skin that is dry (due to a poor or reduced fluid intake) is more susceptible to pressure damage.

When considering the patient's level of mobility, the nurse should consider: activity level, presence of paralysis and restrictions to mobility (e.g. wound drains, intravenous infusions, traction or plaster) and whether these restrictions are temporary or permanent. Patients' general awareness, level of anxiety and the existence of pain should also be assessed.

Assessment of skin should consider whether it is healthy, papery, dry, clammy, sweaty or oedematous. Skin hydration should be noted and any evidence of previous ulceration, sores or broken skin or any pre-existing skin condition or discoloration. Assessing skin with a darker pigmentation needs to be undertaken very carefully, as discoloration tends to be less noticeable.

Patients' continence status should be considered, as incontinence of urine and faeces can lead to skin maceration, and constant washing can remove the natural oils, thus drying the skin.

Medical/surgical history

Patients' previous medical or surgical history will indicate risk factors that impact on tissue perfusion and oxygenation of the tissues. Examples are diabetes, cardiovascular disease and anaemia. Any surgery including the length of time on the operating table, type of anaesthetic (e.g. epidural, spinal, general) should be noted. Medications should be considered, particularly noting antibiotics, steroids, sedatives, anti-inflammatory and cytotoxic drugs or insulin.

Psychological factors

Assessment of patients' emotional status is important (e.g. whether grieving or depressed), as this may affect their motivation.

Lifestyle factors

Whether a patient smokes should be noted, as this may impact on respiratory function. When considering patients' weight and build, a note should be made of whether they are overweight or underweight (see page 110, calculation of body mass index).

Age

The age of the patient should be considered in conjunction with general health. Factors that impact on older patients (nutrition, skin elasticity, the presence of chronic illnesses) may not be significant for those who are younger.

Calculating the risk

Each of the factors above is allocated a score on the chosen assessment tool. The total indicates the level of vulnerability, which in turn should indicate the nature of the prevention plan. However, the allocation of scores for increased vulnerability or elevated risk conditions or behaviours is not consistent across the assessment

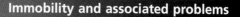

tools. In some, a low total score indicates a high risk of pressure ulcer development, but in others, the opposite is true. There is considerable discussion in the literature as to the advantages and disadvantages of each tool, and the NICE (2005) guidelines suggest that the assessment tool should only be used as an *aide memoire* and should not replace clinical judgement. The risk assessment should be documented in the nursing records along with preventative strategies. The assessment must be repeated at regular intervals or as dictated by any changes in the patient's condition, e.g. following surgery.

PREVENTION OF PRESSURE ULCERS

Principles

Prevention of pressure ulcers will not be achieved unless the predisposing factors are controlled or alleviated for each patient. Generic risk factors were previously identified, but it is the particular combination of these in each patient that determines how high the risk is. Nevertheless, there are general principles to follow when planning preventative strategies.

Careful positioning

Positioning when in bed and sitting in a chair is crucial. All patients who are vulnerable to pressure ulcers should as a minimum be placed on a high-specification (low tech) foam mattresses as they aim to redistribute pressure over a large contact area (NICE 2005). There is little research evidence to suggest that alternating pressure (**Figure 13.1**) or other high-tech pressure-relieving systems are more effective than low-tech devices. However, they should be considered for those patients who are identified as having: a high risk of developing pressure ulcers, a history of pressure damage or a clinical condition that indicates their use, although the effectiveness of the various types is the subject of much debate (NICE 2005).

Regular repositioning

Frequent repositioning is essential whether the patient is in bed or in a chair. A useful yardstick is 2 hours, although this should be adjusted for the individual patient's need. Some patients, particularly those who are elderly, may need to be repositioned more regularly. The repositioning regimen must be rigorously implemented and in some cases can be supported by a repositioning chart, e.g. a 24-hour turning chart.

The use of a pressure-relieving mattress does not remove the need to adjust the patient's position. The 30° tilt is thought to allow pressure to be tolerated for up to three times longer than over bony prominences (Gebhardt 2002c). However, caution needs to be exercised in adopting this approach, as there is conflicting evidence regarding its clinical effectiveness. Bedclothes should be loose and sheets not wrinkled. Pillows can be used to support patients in the desired positions to prevent further deterioration brought about by incorrect positioning of limbs.

When seated in chairs patients should not be left for more than 2 hours regardless of the devices used. The chair must be of appropriate dimensions to promote good posture. There is little evidence that cushions are clinically effective for acutely

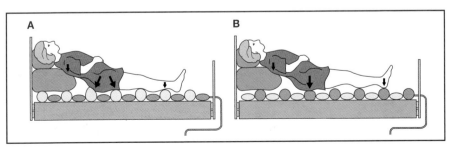

Figure 13.1 Alternating pressure mattress

ill patients, but they may be of some benefit for those who are wheel-chair bound or have a chronic risk of developing pressure ulcers.

Exercise

Passive and active exercise is essential in maintaining and encouraging mobilisation and limiting the impact of some of the predisposing factors.

Safe moving and handling

When moving and handling patients, it is essential that appropriate manual handling equipment is used to prevent shear or friction. Positioning patients to prevent them sliding down the bed is important in preventing shear. The backrest on the hospital bed has been cited as the main culprit in encouraging sliding (Dealey 1999).

Nutrition and hydration

Consideration of patients' nutrition and hydration is important in order to maintain healthy skin and provide assistance with eating and drinking where necessary. Maintaining a food and fluid balance chart may be useful.

Skin care

Continuous assessment of the skin is vital. This can be undertaken when attending to the patient's hygiene needs. Skin should be inspected for persistent erythema, non-blanching hyperaemia, blisters, localised heat, oedema, induration, purplish/bluish localised areas and localised coolness if tissue death occurs. The skin should be kept clean and dry especially if the patient is incontinent, has a high temperature or is sweating excessively. However, caution should be exercised in the overuse of soap and detergents as they are the commonest cause of stripping of the epidermal protective barrier (Butcher 2005). Consideration should be given to the use of non-soap skin cleansers. Emollients in the bath or creams are useful for dry skin and a barrier cream for moist skin may be useful. They do, however, interfere with the use of adhesives on the skin and may also affect the absorptive properties of dressings and continence products (Butcher 2005).

European Pressure Ulcer Advisory Panel Classification System

If the patient does develop a pressure ulcer the European Pressure Ulcer Advisory Panel Classification System should be used to grade it (NICE 2005) (see Table 13.1).

Table 13.1 European Pressure Ulcer Advisory Panel Classification System

Grade 1	Grade 2	Grade 3	Grade 4
Non-blanchable erythema of intact skin. Discoloration of the skin, warmth, oedema, induration or hardness may be used as indicators particularly on individuals with darker skin.	Partial thickness skin loss involving epidermis or dermis or both. The ulcer is superficial and presents clinically as an abrasion or blister.	Full thickness skin loss involving damage to or necrosis of subcutaneous tissue that may extend down to, but not through underlying fascia.	Extensive destruction, tissue necrosis, or damage to muscle, bone or supporting structures with or without full thickness skin loss.

DEEP VEIN THROMBOSIS

Preparation

Patient	Equipment/Environment	Nurse
• Patients who are immobile, undergoing surgery or have a predisposing factor are at risk of developing deep vein thrombosis (DVT). • Dehydration and hypotension increase the risk.	• Tape measure. • Anti-embolism stockings of appropriate size and length (calf or knee length) **PFP1**.	• The hands should be clean and an apron worn. • Additional protective clothing may be necessary if indicated by the patient's condition (see Chapter 9).

Procedure

1. Early mobilisation, if the patient's condition allows, reduces the risk of deep vein thrombosis (DVT).

2. Teach the patient foot and leg exercises before an operation or period of immobility and encourage exercises at least hourly. Position the patient's legs on the theatre table or in bed so as to prevent calf compression. Discourage the patient from crossing the legs in bed.

3. If the patient is unable to do foot and leg exercises, the nurse or physiotherapist should perform passive leg movements.

4. Deep breathing should be encouraged.

5. Observe the calves for swelling, heat and tenderness. If DVT is present, the calf may appear paler in colour than the calf of the other leg.

6. Measure the legs according to the manufacturer's instructions.

7. Fit the anti-embolic stockings according to the manufacturer's instructions (Figure 13.2).

8. Subcutaneous heparin or clexane may be prescribed as a prophylactic measure.

Post procedure

Patient	Equipment/Environment	Nurse
• Encourage the patient to carry out leg movements and avoid activities that may increase the risk of DVT (e.g. crossing legs).	• Remove anti-embolism stockings at least once daily, to inspect the skin and calves. • Check frequently that the stockings are not wrinkled or rolled down.	• Document the potential problem and nursing actions on the care plan.

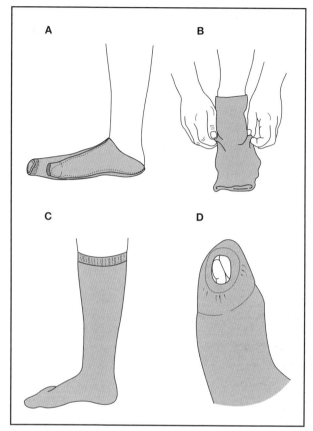

Figure 13.2 Fitting anti-embolism stockings

Points for practice

1. Thigh-length stockings can be more difficult to apply and may not be as effective if the thigh and calf are not in proportion; the stocking may be too tight or too loose in one area (Byrne 2002). The type required will be prescribed by the doctor. Anti-embolism stockings work by promoting venous flow in the legs and preventing stasis (Hayes et al 2002).

References and further reading

Moving and handling

Royal College of Nursing. (2003) *Manual handling assessment in hospital and the community: an RCN guide*. RCN Revised, London.

> Provides practical advice on risk assessment in moving and handling. Available on the website www.rcn.org.uk.

Smith J (ed.) (2005). *The guide to the handling of people*, 5th edn. Back Care, Teddington, Middlesex.

> This is the latest edition of 'The guide to the handling of patients' published by Back Care in association with the RCN and National Back Exchange. It is widely recognised as the most comprehensive resource available for moving and handling.

Pressure ulcers

Butcher M. (2005) Prevention and management of superficial pressure ulcers. *British Journal of Community Nursing* 10(6 Suppl):S16, S18–S20.

> This article examines superficial pressure ulcers, those involving the upper layers of the skin. The article presents a practical approach for nurses in preventing pressure damage with a strong emphasis on skin care and reduction of friction.

Dealey C. (1999) *The care of wounds*, 2nd edn. Blackwell, London.

> This book addresses all aspects of wound care management including pressure ulcers.

Gebhardt K. (2002a) Prevention of pressure ulcers – Part 1 Causes of pressure ulcers. *Nursing Times* 98(11):41–44.

> The first in a series of three articles examines the causes of pressure ulcers.

Gebhardt K. (2002b) Prevention of pressure ulcers – Part 2 Patient assessment. *Nursing Times* 98(12):39–42.

> This second article in the series outlines how the incidence of pressure ulcers can be kept to a minimum by identifying patients who have an elevated risk. This article focuses on a range of factors associated with assessment.

Gebhardt K. (2002c) Prevention of pressure ulcers – Part 3 Prevention strategies. *Nursing Times* 98(13):37–40.

> Although aspects of the debate have now been superseded by the NICE clinical guideline 29, this article outlines the benefits and limitation of the tools used to assess pressure ulcers and the aids used for pressure relief. Areas for further research are identified.

Norton D, McLaren R, Exton-Smith A. (1975) *An investigation of geriatric nursing problems in hospital*. Churchill Livingstone, Edinburgh.

> This is the original research that led to the development of the first pressure ulcer risk assessment tool, the Norton score designed to be used with elderly patients.

Russell L. (2002) Pressure ulcer classification: the systems and the pitfalls. *British Journal of Nursing* 11(12 Suppl):S49–S59.

> This article provides an overview of the various classification systems used in the grading of pressure ulcers. Included is an outline of the European Pressure Ulcer Advisory Panel Classification System, which is now recommended by NICE.

Thompson D. (2005) An evaluation of the Waterlow pressure ulcer risk-assessment tool. *British Journal of Nursing* 14(8):455–458.

> This article reviews studies related to the reliability and validity of the Waterlow pressure ulcer risk-assessment tool and concludes that whilst it has not been developed on scientific principles, it

is a useful and practical way of systematically evaluating and re-evaluating individual patients' vulnerability to developing pressure ulcers.

Waterlow J. (2005) From costly treatment to cost-effective prevention: using Waterlow. *British Journal of Community Nursing* **10**(9 Suppl):S25–S30.

This is an updated article outlining the use of the Waterlow pressure ulcer risk-assessment tool. Waterlow describes the recent update to the system and explains how pressure-ulcer risk assessments should be undertaken.

Deep vein thrombosis

Byrne B. (2002) Deep vein thrombosis prophylaxis: the effectiveness and implications of using below knee or thigh length graduated compression stockings. *Heart & Lung: The Journal of Acute and Critical Care* **30**(4):277–284.

This article reviews the literature available to support the use of below-knee or thigh-length stockings. It starts with a nice overview of the risk factors for DVT and also explains how external compression devices and graduated compression stockings work and the importance of correct measurement and careful application.

Geraghty S, Russell J, Gilbourne S, Young J. (2001) Deep vein thrombosis – aetiology and prevention. *Nursing Times* **97**(17):34–35.

This article gives an overview of the causes of DVT and how they can be prevented. Good photographs showing how to measure and fit below-knee graded compressions stockings.

National Institute of Clinical Excellence. (2007) *Venous thromboembolism (deep vein thrombosis and pulmonary embolus) in surgical patients.* NICE, London. www.nice.org.uk.

This provides guidance on the prevention and management of DVT and pulmonary embolus in adults undergoing a range of surgical procedures.

Wallis M, Autar R. (2001) Deep vein thrombosis: clinical nursing management. *Nursing Standard* **15**(18):47–54.

Websites

European Pressure Ulcer Advisory Panel. (2003) *Pressure Ulcer Prevention Guidelines.* Available at www.epuap.org.uk.

National Institute Clinical Excellence (NICE). (2005) *The prevention and treatment of pressure ulcers (Clinical Guideline 29).* NICE, London. Available at www.nice.org.uk.

Royal College of Nursing. (2001) *Pressure ulcer risk assessment and prevention – clinical practice guidelines.* RCN, London. Available at www.rcn.org.uk.

Notes